— Bailliè
Handbook

GW00633916

— Baillière's ——————
Handbook of First Aid

Revised by

Norman G. Kirby
OBE, OStJ, FRCS, FRCS(Ed), FICS
Major-General, late RAMC
Accident and Emergency Unit
Guy's Hospital, London

and

Stephen J. Mather
MB, BS, LRCP, MRCS, DRCOG, FFARCS (Eng.)
Department of Anaesthetics
Bristol Royal Infirmary
Bristol

Seventh Edition

Baillière Tindall London Philadelphia Toronto
Mexico City Rio de Janeiro Sydney Tokyo Hong Kong

Baillière Tindall 1 St Anne's Road
W. B. Saunders   Eastbourne, East Sussex BN21 3UN, England

West Washington Square
Philadelphia, PA 19105, USA

1 Goldthorne Avenue
Toronto, Ontario M8Z 5T9, Canada

Apartado 26370 — Cedro 512
Mexico 4, DF Mexico

Rua Evaristo da Veiga 55,20° andar
Rio de Janeiro — RJ, Brazil

ABP Australia Ltd, 44–50 Waterloo Road
North Ryde, NSW 2113, Australia

Ichibancho Central Building, 22–1 Ichibancho
Chiyoda-ku, Tokyo 102, Japan

10/fl, Inter-Continental Plaza, 94 Granville Road
Tsim Sha Tsui East, Kowloon, Hong Kong

First published 1941
Sixth edition 1970
 Reprinted 1975
Seventh edition 1985

Typeset by Photo·Graphics, Honiton, Devon
Printed in Great Britain by Biddles Ltd of Guildford Surrey

British Library Cataloguing in Publication Data
Kirby, Norman G.
 Baillière's handbook of first aid.——7th ed.
 1. First aid in illness and injury
 I. Title   II. Mather, Stephen J.
 616.02'52   RC87

ISBN 0–7020–1097–9

Contents

Preface, vii

Part 1 Assessment of the Casualty and Emergency Response

1 Assessment of the Casualty, 3
2 Action at a Road Traffic Accident, 8
3 Mass Casualties, 11
4 Emotional Response to Disaster, 14
5 Cardiopulmonary Resuscitation, 16
6 Pregnancy and Emergency Childbirth, 23

Part 2 Structure and Function

7 Cells, Tissues and Organs, 33
8 The Respiratory System, 36
9 The Heart and Circulation, 41
10 The Nervous System and Sense Organs, 47
11 The Skeleton, 59
12 Joints and the Muscular System, 73
13 The Digestive System, 78
14 Foodstuffs, Metabolism and Body Temperature, 83

Part 3 Clinical Practice

15 Asphyxia and Respiratory Disorders, 91
16 Cardiac and Circulatory Problems, 107
17 The Abdomen, 118
18 Wounds and their Treatment, 122
19 Wound Infections, 131
20 Fractures, 134
21 Injuries to the Joints and Muscles, 180

vi Contents

22 Spinal Injuries, 191
23 Sports Injuries, 202
24 Unconsciousness – General Principles, 211
25 Head, Brain and Facial Injury, 217
26 Medical Causes of Unconsciousness, 230
27 The Effects of Temperature, 241
28 Poisons, 246
29 Psychogenic Ailments, 254
30 Burns, 258
31 Nuclear Disasters, Chemical and Biological Warfare, 264
32 Disorders of the Eye, Ear and Nose, 271
33 Bites and Stings, 279
34 Bandaging, Dressing and Roller Bandage Techniques, 282
35 Transport of the Sick and Injured, 317
36 Transport by Stretcher, 329

Index, 353

Preface

First aid is, like medicine, both an art and a science. Interest and some natural ability are necessary, but more fundamental is the need to learn the basic principles thoroughly, to revise, keep up to date, and look for new ideas.

There have always been a large number of public-minded citizens who have learnt and practised life saving aid; a few notable examples are the St John Ambulance Association and Brigade, the British Red Cross Society, the St Andrew's Ambulance Association, the police, ambulance and fire services, and members of the youth organizations (the Boys' Brigade, the Boy Scouts and the Girl Guides). However, members of these groups will not always be present, and there is a need for more general, widespread teaching. We would recommend, for example, the teaching of first aid at schools, during the day and in the evening.

This book is intended for instructors and for those who will practise advanced first aid: nurses, medical students, members of the voluntary aid societies, and the police, ambulance and fire services.

Baillière's Handbook of First Aid has been revised extensively for this new edition. Dr John Henry, MRCP, Consultant Physician to the National Poisons Information Unit, Guy's Hospital, has kindly revised the section on poisoning, and Dr Tanya Malpass, MRCP, DCH, Senior Registrar, Accident and Emergency Department, Guy's Hospital, has revised the medical emergencies.

We have divided the book into three main parts:

Assessment of the Casualty and Emergency Response. The essential principles of emergency first aid have not changed over the years, but the emphasis has. Cardiopulmonary resuscitation, CPR, has been brought to the forefront. The full importance of those first four minutes has been well established: the need for urgent attention to airway, breathing, bleeding and circulation is now widely recognized. The basic principles of this life saving technique have been simplified and standardized.

Structure and Function. A good background knowledge of human anatomy and physiology adds interest and expertise to life saving aid, and we have therefore revised the section on this. This will be of sufficient detail for instructors.

Clinical Practice. The newer materials used in dressings have been looked at. Members of the London Ambulance Service advised us on the lifting and carrying of patients and stretchers: the time-honoured procedures and methods have not changed.

The production of the manuscript has involved a lot of typing and re-typing, and we would like to thank Mrs Caroline Dean, Mrs Celia Mather, and Mrs Cynthia Kirby for the clear copies they have made from our notes and dictation. The staff from Baillière Tindall have cajoled and guided us through the difficulties of producing a manuscript for publication, and we would like to thank Mr David Dickens, Editorial Director, Mrs Elizabeth K. E. Bridger, and Mr Graham Smith for their help, advice and encouragement at crucial times. Dr Brian Robertson, MRCS, LRCP, and Dr P. J. F. Baskett, MB, BCh, BAO, FFARCS, of the British Association for Immediate Care, read the final script and made many useful suggestions. Miss Anne McGuinness, FRCS (Ed), Registrar in the Accident and Emergency Department of Guy's Hospital, read the galley proofs.

We would also like to point out that, although the pronoun 'he' has been used throughout the book, this is merely a literary convention. It should be understood to mean 'he or she' in all cases.

We hope that this book will continue to stimulate, educate and guide all those who render aid to the sick and injured in emergencies.

Norman G. Kirby
Stephen J. Mather

Part 1
Assessment of the Casualty and Emergency Response

— 1

Assessment of the Casualty

Approach to the incident

First aiders must always consider their own safety. Often the inexperienced or unthinking, in the heat of the moment, put themselves at greater risk. Making sure of his own safety the first aider should approach the incident prepared to take charge if necessary. Bystanders, if any, can assist by going for help; if there are two they can be sent in opposite directions. In road traffic accidents the emergency services should be contacted first by dialling 999 (in the UK) and told

1. Location, road number, grid reference, landmarks.
2. Type of accident.
3. Number of vehicles involved.
4. Number of casualties
5. Any casualties trapped.
6. Special hazards – fire, chemical spillage, etc.

The aim of any treatment, whoever it is given by, is to prevent an existing condition deteriorating and provide, as far as is possible in the circumstances, the best conditions for recovery.

The first essential in approaching an incident is to avoid panic. This applies to all involved, the first aider and through him the casualty and bystanders. This means that the first aider must have a calm and reassuring manner, even if he does not feel calm and reassured himself. By adopting this attitude a crisis situation is often defused and the first aid given that much more effective.

Assessing the incident

A rapid assessment of the situation and a note of the number of casualties is first made. Each casualty should be looked at individually and an order of priority decided. There is a danger that the first casualty met with is the first to be treated; this attitude is not unnatural, but ignores the possibility that the second or third may be more severely injured. A mistaken order of priorities can be as dangerous as no first aid treatment being available at all. The casualty who is clamouring for attention may be in less danger than a silent motionless one.

3

Priorities

Airway problems and major bleeding always take precedence over fractures, minor wounds and hysteria.

The first aider must check that each casualty
(a) has an adequate airway,
(b) is breathing,
(c) has no major bleeding, and
(d) is conscious.

If the answer to all of these is 'yes', he can be left in the care of a bystander. If the first aider is alone, each casualty will have to be left until all have been assessed.

Once this has been done it is necessary to decide who needs most help. This may not be the most seriously injured – a person who has been knocked out and only requires airway support will have his life saved by simple treatment given in time. The first aider may find it impossible to do anything effective for a casualty with severe multiple injuries.

Spinal injuries

If a spinal injury is suspected, it is best not to move the casualty until professional help arrives, unless he is in immediate danger from, for example, fire or imminent building collapse. This does not preclude attention to the airway or bleeding, which need not change the position in which the casualty is found.

Unconscious casualties

They should be placed in the recovery position (Fig. 1.1). If available, a bystander can be asked to hold the jaw forward to maintain an open airway (see Fig. 5.2) and monitor pulse and respiration.

Bystanders

Many people feel helpless in the face of an accident, but many also want to assist. Bystanders can be used to control traffic, get help and do specific tasks, e.g. apply pressure to a wound in a case of haemorrhage. By using bystanders in this way, their feelings of wanting to help can be employed to best advantage. The first aider can then be free to give his attention to the total situation.

Working alone

The lone first aider with one or more casualties should use the same guidelines as outlined above. Having assessed the incident, he will have to

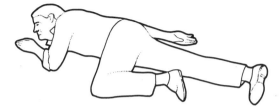

Fig. 1.1 The recovery position. If there are major limb fractures turn the casualty on his side and support him with pillows, rolled blankets or coats, without moving the limbs more than is necessary.

decide whether to treat any or all before summoning help. In remote situations there may be the added problem of having to wait until rescued. It is vital that the first aider remain calm and think logically.

Most first aid treatment is common sense.

Clothes and protective headgear

In many accidents, particularly road accidents, the injury will necessitate the removal of some of the casualty's clothes to make an effective assessment. Motorcyclists, for example, may have to have their helmets removed if there are airway problems, vomiting or severe bleeding from the head and neck. When removing the crash helmet it is advisable for the head and neck to be supported by an assistant.

Clothes that are not easily removable without disturbing the casualty unduly – for example, in cases of fracture – may be slit along the seams. Clothes which cover an injured part should never be tugged at repeatedly.

Remember that extreme gentleness is required at all times.

Examination of the casualty

First check that the airway is adequate. Breathing which is noisy, sounding as though the casualty is snoring, means the airway is at least partially obstructed. Make sure he is breathing adequately (look at the chest – is it expanding? Feel for breath on the hand) and that he has a pulse. Adults breathe about 16 times a minute, babies about 30–40 times a minute. In the same way the pulse rate varies with age, from 140 per minute at birth to around 60–80 in the adult. Remember the pulse rate will rise in shock states (see Chapter 3) and when there is pain. Check for any characteristic smell on the breath (e.g. acetone in diabetic coma).

Look at the casualty's colour. Cyanosis may indicate asphyxia. This may be due to the inhalation of vomit, teeth or dentures. Check that the mouth is empty. Full dentures may be left in the mouth only if the airway cannot be supported without them. As a good general rule, however, such a potentially dangerous foreign body should be removed.

Check for bleeding from the ear and nose. Leakage of clear or straw-coloured fluid from them may indicate a fractured skull.

Examine the pupils carefully. Do they get smaller on exposure to bright light (on opening the lid or on shining a torch in the eye)? When his eyelash is touched gently the casualty should blink. Check for any bleeding on the white of the eye – the eye will look bloodshot.

Feel the scalp below the hair and note any lacerations. Occasionally a fracture of the skull can be felt through a wound.

Feel the contour of the cervical spine (the vertebrae of the neck). Is the contour smooth? If the casualty is conscious find out if there is any pain in the neck or any tenderness when finger pressure is applied over the bones. If there is, or if a neck injury is suspected, a cervical collar (see Fig. 22.7) should be applied. In emergencies one can be made from a rolled-up newspaper bandaged round the neck.

Examine next the chest and the rest of the spine. Check that both sides of the chest move to the same extent with each breath. Look for any penetrating injuries or 'sucking wounds' (see Fig. 15.7). Make a note of any tender spots over the rib cage. If the airway is obstructed there will be an indrawing of the soft tissues between the ribs and under the rib margins. This is especially common in children. Examine the spine in the same way as the neck. If the casualty is supine this can be done by sliding a hand under the back. If at all possible, do not move a casualty with a spinal injury. If resuscitation is required, repositioning may be unavoidable. In this situation the casualty should be moved 'in one piece' with the aid of several helpers.

Check the pelvic area by gently exerting pressure on both sides at the same time, so as to slightly compress the pelvic ring. Any sign of tenderness should lead one to suspect a fracture. Incontinence may be the result of fright, unconsciousness or a pelvic fracture.

Examine the abdomen for wounds and bruising. Bowel may protrude from abdominal wounds.

Examine the limbs in turn for any swelling, deformity or major bleeding. Note the shape and size of joints compared with the opposite side. Bleeding into a joint may result in profound swelling and severe pain. Remember that blood loss into limb fractures may be considerable and that there may be no external evidence of bleeding, the only signs being swelling over the fracture site, pain and shock.

Check for any warning medallions such as Medic-Alert around the wrist or neck. They can alert one to a particular condition or drug therapy, particularly steroids. There may be injection marks on the thighs or abdomen of diabetics. Drug addicts may have injection marks on the arms or, more rarely, legs.

Assess the level of consciousness in every casualty. Particularly note if he is becoming more or less responsive.

Conscious level is best assessed by noting
  (a)   eye opening
  (b)   purposeful movement
  (c)   spoken response
following these stimuli:
  (a)   spoken word
  (b)   touch
  (c)   pain (pinching the skin).
Test also for the eyelash reflex – touch the lash, it should cause blinking.

Remember that in spinal injury the casualty may be unable to feel below the level of the injury yet may be fully conscious. In this case, touch and pinch him on the leg; if there is no response, move up the body until he can feel the stimulus.

Remember that fractures in the neck may also lead to difficulty with respiration.

It is vital to write down all these observations on paper, with the times at which they were made. Any history from the casualty or bystanders should also be recorded.

Further information

Always check through the pockets, handbag or luggage of an unconscious patient; this is best done in the presence of a witness. Look for information cards which indicate if the casualty is diabetic or on steroids. Look for hospital or GP's appointments cards, blood group cards, tablets, medicines, insulin or sugar.

Reassurance

The single most important principle is **first, do no harm**. Be gentle but methodical. Your casualty must have confidence in his rescuer. **Reassurance** is sometimes the most effective treatment one can give. No matter what the injury, the patient must be reassured that he is in good hands and that help is on its way. It is important to repeat this over and over again, since anxiety will certainly not improve the patient's condition, and may actually make him worse.

2

Action at a Road Traffic Accident

Road traffic accidents are increasing in number and in severity. With the development of high-speed motorways, multiple collisions and involvements are becoming more common, particularly in times of reduced visibility, fog, or torrential rain. Cars rapidly lose control by skidding on smooth surfaces such as ice and by aquaplaning on water.

When confronted with a road traffic accident you must first carefully assess the situation to make sure that you and your car are visible and not at risk of being hit by another vehicle. Pull well away from the traffic stream if possible, as many 'samaritans' have been killed or severely injured.

Assess the position of the cars in the accident, turn off ignition and ensure no smoking, particularly if there is a smell of fuel. Detach the batteries if necessary. Check the airway of any people who are injured, unconscious or trapped. Blood, vomit, or dentures may need to be cleared, and the position of the patient's head should be adjusted carefully to improve air entry. Quickly examine the patient, assessing fractures, shock and wounds. If there is excessive bleeding, treat this by the application of a firm pad and bandage, with supplementary splintage if necessary.

If the patient is trapped in the seat, leave him alone unless he is in danger from fire or further damage. Send for assistance rapidly to the fire and ambulance services. It is important to inform the ambulance service that the casualties are trapped or there is some other serious hazard, because in some areas of the UK the ambulance service can call on appropriately equipped and trained doctors to attend the scenes of accidents. This may be a hospital-based flying squad or volunteer immediate care doctors belonging to Schemes affiliated to the British Association for Immediate Care (BASICS). This saves time and improves the patients' chance of recovery.

Attempts should be made to count the passengers, as quite often passengers are thrown from the car and may travel several yards landing behind hedges or in ditches. Children may be lying on the floor of the car and should be looked for. On the whole, it is better to leave trapped patients in the vehicle until the emergency services arrive unless there is considerable risk, in which case swift action should be taken with as many people as possible to move the patient rapidly and steadily, preferably after applying splints. In this situation be careful of the cervical and thoracic spine; move the patient 'in one piece', using as many of the bystanders as possible. He should then be placed in a position of safety; if unconscious in the recovery position, otherwise on his back. If he has a chest injury, he may be more comfortable sitting up.

What happened

History:
From the patient
From bystanders
(Note damage to vehicles which may give clues to the type of injury to be expected. Count all casualties. Is anyone known to be missing?)

What does the casualty feel? (symptoms)

Pain
Breathlessness
Loss of normal sensation
Nausea
Faintness
Disorientation
Loss of memory
For events before the incident
For events after the incident
Thirst ⎫
Palpitations ⎬ These may indicate bleeding
Cold, clammy skin ⎭

Information gained by examination (signs)

Adequacy of:
Airway
Breathing
Circulation (and control of bleeding)
Colour
Conscious level
Eyelash reflex
Swelling
Deformity
Bruising
Tenderness
Incontinence
Temperature

Outside factors

Observe:
The weather – hot, cold, rain, snow
The environment – rural, urban, remote
Hazards – chemicals, toxic gases, fire risks

— 3

Mass Casualties

A mass casualty situation occurs when the medical resources of an area are overwhelmed or about to be overwhelmed by some incident, with no immediate prospect of outside assistance.

Incidents which can lead to mass casualties occurring can be divided into three:
1. Natural – flood, earthquake, etc.
2. Transport – road, rail, air, sea.
3. Man-made – Deliberate: war, terrorist activity.
              – Accident: industry, mines, etc.

From this definition it will be seen that first aid in such a situation can decide the chances of the injured's survival and the quality of recovery. Skilled first aid is the first line of treatment, and the first aider will often have to assess the priorities (triage – Fig. 3.1).

The first aider faced with mass casualties has to:
(a) do as little as possible,
(b) keep what is done simple, and
(c) do it quickly to as many as possible.

Triage is the term given to casualty sorting, by which priority of treatment and removal from the scene are assessed. In war it means arranging care for those who will most benefit.

Assessment of priorities for evacuation

The rapid evacuation of casualties who require surgical treatment is vital in reducing the mortality of the wounded. However, not all casualties need to be evacuated and a proportion, after receiving treatment, will be fit to return to their homes or to their work.

Those casualties who require evacuation must be sorted into priorities based on their need for surgery and/or resuscitation. The following classification is used, priority one cases being those requiring most urgent evacuation.

Priority One: cases requiring resuscitation and early surgery

Respiratory emergencies:
1. Asphyxia due to respiratory obstruction.
2. Maxillofacial wounds with established or imminent asphyxia.

11

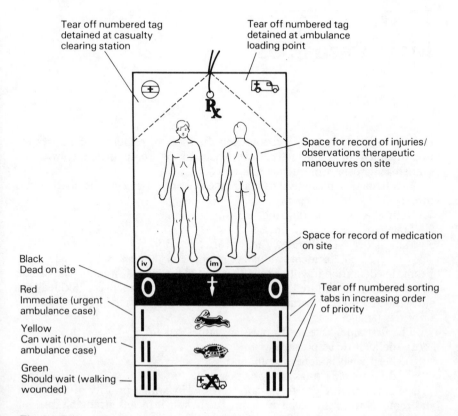

Fig. 3.1 Triage label. Courtesy of Loxley Medical.

3. Sucking wounds of chest.
4. Tension pneumothorax.

Shock due to:
1. Major haemorrhage from visceral injuries, cardio-pericardial injuries or wounds with massive muscle damage.
2. Multiple wounds and major fractures.
3. Severe burns – over 20% body surface burnt.

Priority Two: cases requiring early surgery and possible resuscitation

1. Penetrating abdominal wounds; visceral injuries, including perforations of the gastrointestinal tract; wounds of the genitourinary tract and thoracic injuries without asphyxia.

2. Major vessel injuries requiring repair.
3. Brain and spinal injuries, open or closed, requiring decompression.
4. Burns – under 20% body surface burnt in certain locations, e.g. face, hands, feet, genitalia and perineum.

Priority Three

1. All other brain and spinal injuries.
2. Soft tissue injuries requiring wound toilet.
3. Lesser fractures and dislocations.
4. Eye injuries.
5. Maxillofacial injuries without asphyxia.
6. Burns of other locations – under 20% body surface burnt.

It is essential to recognize that casualty sorting is a dynamic and not a static process. Many factors affect a decision. A significant alteration in one of them may allow the patient to be placed in a new category.

Once the priorities have been established, the normal principles and practices of first aid should be employed.

4

Emotional Response to Disaster

The varying emotional response of individuals to disasters is recognized as an uncontrollable factor in disaster planning. Not everyone knows how they will behave under stress, despite constant planning and training. Because of the nature of disasters people make mistakes and errors of judgement, and defects are revealed in even the best worked-out plans. Well-trained, well-motivated teams who have worked together for some time are most effective, and less prone to emotional problems. It is important to realize that fear is a natural tendency and that everyone will feel this to some degree. The common manifestations are trembling, sweating and fast pulse, possibly with loss of bowel or bladder control.

Immediately after a disaster occurs, people are temporarily unable to cope with the situation. There is rarely panic, but one will see that people are dazed, apathetic, stunned and under stress. Slowly they will begin to look after themselves and extricate themselves from damage, then they will start to look for members of the family. However, this will probably be largely uncontrolled, e.g. using hands instead of tools. At this stage they will welcome help and some form of active control. People are very adaptable to disaster and it is surprising how the degree of control improves.

After this initial phase, a certain number of people will become excitable, quick-tempered and aggressive. They are dissatisfied and difficult to control, and unfortunately tend to aggravate others. They feel that something must be done: the obvious remedy is to give them something purposeful to do.

It must also be remembered that trained people working long hours under difficult conditions and danger will, in addition to the fatigue which is normally experienced, develop exhaustion. This may show itself by unexpected changes in behaviour, excessive talkativeness, and indecision. There may be severe apprehension, restlessness, an over-reaction to sound, and trembling. Various physical symptoms such as weakness or deafness may appear. It is important that this state is recognized and that the patient is made to rest and immediately taken away from the difficult situation. After rest and sleep, they are often fit to come back again.

Treatment

Immediately after a disaster, people will require active reassurance. They must be convinced that something positive is being done to help them and

14

their families. The sooner they can be restored to the family group the better: the preservation of the family is important. The ability to give good, accurate information whenever possible will also help. Rehabilitation of people in this state of emotional shock is achieved by making them carry out some useful activity. They will accept guidance, be cooperative, and will readily do useful work at the scene. Being given the opportunity to talk over their experience with other people involved will also speed their recovery. At all times, be confident that this condition is merely a passing phase and that the vast majority of people make a full recovery from emotional shock.

5

Cardiopulmonary Resuscitation (Heart–lung Resuscitation)

Principle

The casualty is no longer breathing for himself or has inadequate circulation. In this situation, the oxygen supply to the tissues will be cut off. The brain is most at risk and will be irreversibly damaged after a few minutes.

Effective resuscitation should achieve 'ABC':

A. A clear AIRWAY
B. Restoration of BREATHING
C. Adequate CIRCULATION

Resuscitation may consist of simply opening an obstructed airway, or full mouth to mouth artificial respiration and cardiac massage to assist the circulation.

The airway

The commonest causes of obstruction are:

The tongue falling back in the throat of an unconscious casualty and blocking the airway (this is the most common).

An inhaled foreign body, usually food in adults, peanuts and small objects in children.

Blood or vomit after an injury.

To open the obstructed airway (Fig. 5.1):

1. Lift the jaw forward.
2. Tilt the head back on the neck.
3. Attempt to remove any foreign body with the fingers.

This in itself may relieve the obstruction. If it does not, recourse may be had to back blows or the Heimlich manoeuvre (page 94). If breathing starts again spontaneously, turn the casualty into the recovery position **but continue to support the airway by holding the chin forward.** If respiration does not recommence spontaneously, artificial respiration must be started without delay. The use of the Brook airway is more effective, less unpleasant and removes the fear of infection (see Fig. 5.2).

16

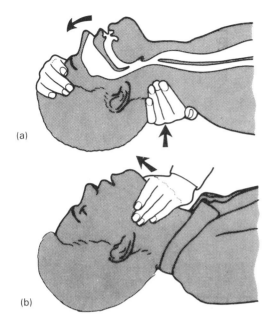

(a)

Fig. 5.1(a) Tilt the head back upon the neck (which is slightly flexed by the hand placed under it). Arrows show the direction of movement.

(b)

Fig. 5.1(b) The open airway is maintained by holding the chin forwards and upwards.

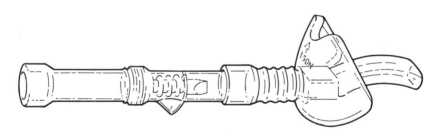

Fig. 5.2 The Brook airway.

Breathing

First check that the airway is not simply obstructed again. Active breathing movements against an obstructed airway will cause indrawing of the soft tissues above between and below the ribs. This is especially easy to see in children. Listen at the mouth, or feel for breath with your hand or your cheek, or look for condensation on a mirror held close to the casualty's mouth. The most common causes of respiratory arrest are:

(a) obstructed airway
(b) cardiac arrest
(c) severe shock
(d) chest trauma
(e) head injury
(f) electrocution
(g) stroke
(h) poisoning
(i) drowning.

Such patients look pale and blue.

No matter what the cause, the same action must be taken – artificial respiration.

Artificial respiration by the expired air method

1. Ensure an open airway, as above.
2. Turn the casualty onto his back.
3. Kneeling by his side, pinch the nose with one hand while lifting his chin forward with the other.
4. Take a large breath and place your own mouth completely over that of the casualty. *A good seal is essential.* 'Mouth to nose' techniques should be used with children, or 'mouth to mouth-and-nose' with babies.
5. Blow to inflate the casualty's lungs; this may be harder than you think.
6. Look for movement of the chest wall as you blow. It should expand to its normal extent.
7. Take your mouth away and feel for the casualty's exhaled breath on your cheek; watch the chest fall.

If the chest does not rise, either
(a) the airway is still obstructed, or
(b) there was an imperfect seal between your own mouth and that of the casualty.

Expired air respiration is useless unless the chest expands.

After about six breaths, check to see if the casualty has started breathing again. Vomiting may occur at this stage, and one may have to turn the casualty quickly into the recovery position. Respiration is inadequate if
(a) it is very shallow, or
(b) it is very slow (less than 10 breaths per minute in the adult, 15–20 in children, 25–30 in babies).

Respiratory arrest may quickly lead to cardiac arrest; prompt treatment is essential.

Circulation

If the heart has stopped, or the circulation is inadequate, combined cardiopulmonary (heart–lung) resuscitation (CPR) is required. Such patients are usually pale or blue, pulseless and unconscious. Causes of cardiac arrest are:

    (a) heart attack
    (b) abnormal heart rhythm (irregular pulse)
    (c) severe haemorrhage
    (d) electrocution
    (e) head injury
    (f) chest injury
    (g) respiratory arrest
    (h) poisoning.

Whatever the cause, treatment is the same – CPR.

Cardiopulmonary resuscitation comprises:
1. Expired air respiration (EAR)
2. Chest compression (closed chest cardiac massage or CCCM)
Expired air respiration is performed as above. Four inflations of the lungs are given prior to starting chest compression. **To perform chest compression adequately, the casualty must be laid on a hard surface.**

Whilst assessing the casualty, any major bleeding must be stopped. This is essential for an efficient circulation.
Proceed as follows:
1. Locate the breast bone (sternum) by feeling for the notch where the collar bones meet (upper end) and the angle formed between the rib margins (lower end) (Fig. 5.3).
2. Place the heel of one hand over the lower third of the sternum and place the other hand upon the first (make sure the finger tips do not press onto the ribs, which can easily be fractured). In this position the hands lie over the heart (Fig. 5.4).
3. **Keeping the arms straight**, rock forwards to compress the casualty's chest about 5 cm (2 inches) in an adult. This should bring the arms vertically above the casualty's chest. Rocking backwards and forwards alternately releases and compresses the heart, forcing blood around the circulation. This rocking motion is less tiring than might be expected and can be maintained for long periods of time.

    Children require much less pressure. In children aged 5–10 years only one hand should be used, compressing the chest 2.5 cm (1 inch). In babies **only two fingers** are required, the depth of compression being 1.5–2 cm (approximately half to three-quarters of an inch).

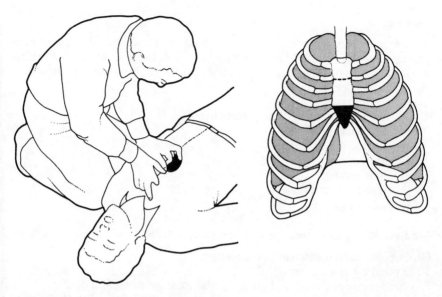

Fig. 5.3 Locating the lower third of the sternum.

Rate of compression

This must not be too fast or the heart will not have time to fill between each 'beat'. In adults the rate should be 60 per minute. If working alone, the rate should be rather more than one per second, to allow for ventilation at a rate of two breaths per fifteen compressions.

In children the rates should be 80–100 compressions per minute, with two breaths for each fifteen compressions. If there are two rescuers, compressions should be carried out continuously; it is not necessary to stop for ventilation, the breath being given on relaxing from the fifth compression.

Babies should receive compression rates of 120 per minute or more if possible. The ventilation rate for babies will remain at about 12 per minute, as it is difficult in practice to exceed this number whilst providing an adequate heart rate.

Remember, cardiopulmonary resuscitation demands both expired air respiration and cardiac massage.

If the casualty's heartbeat resumes, *he may still require artificial ventilation*. Only when both spontaneous breathing and pulses are adequate should he be turned into the recovery position. If he is unconscious, the airway must be supported. Successful resuscitation should result in an improvement in the

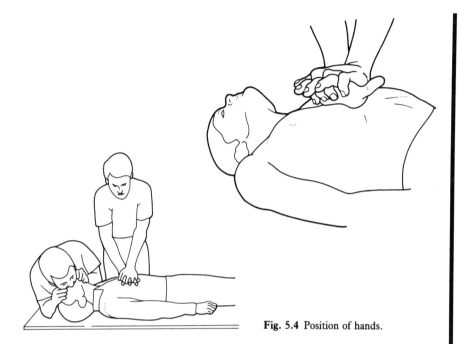

Fig. 5.4 Position of hands.

colour of the patient as normal circulation is restored, and an improvement in the level of consciousness (although full orientation with the surroundings may not be achieved).
In summary,

Successful resuscitation will achieve ABC:
A. an open AIRWAY
B. restoration of BREATHING
C. adequate CIRCULATION

Resuscitation in difficult circumstances

In certain circumstances it may be difficult or impossible to perform resuscitation as outlined above due, for example, to the casualty being trapped in a sitting position or face down. However, even under these conditions cardiac massage **can** still be performed effectively against a hard surface and should be attempted if at all possible.

Resuscitation must take priority over all other injuries and if necessary the casualty should be moved to allow resuscitation to be performed.

Artificial ventilation by the expired air method may be difficult if there are severe facial injuries or repeated vomiting, but it is by no means impossible. If facial injuries prevent a good seal around the mouth, a pad or dressing should be used to complete the seal and prevent leakage of air in so far as is practicable. Foreign bodies, vomit or blood clot must be removed with the fingers.

Artificial ventilation should always be attempted, even if success seems remote.

In very exceptional and infrequent cases, artificial ventilation by the expired air method may be impossible because either
(a)   the patient cannot physically be moved because he is trapped, or
(b)   he is contaminated with a dangerous chemical (for example organophosphorus insecticide) which may put the rescuer's own life at risk.
A decision then has to be made whether to wait for the Emergency Services or to perform a 'manual' method of artificial ventilation, such as the Holger–Nielsen technique. Artificial ventilation alone may restore the heartbeat in some cases and should be tried even if cardiac massage is impossible.

No other method of artificial ventilation is as effective as EAR and this should always be used if practicable.

It is quite possible to give EAR to a casualty sitting up or even lying semi-prone, provided the face can be reached.

The Holger–Nielsen technique

This is suitable for those trapped face down, **when neither EAR nor cardiac massage can be used.**
1. The face should be turned to one side and the airway opened. If there are two rescuers, one should maintain the open airway by lifting the jaw forward. Place the casualty's arms so that his hands are clasped under his head.
2. Kneel astride the casualty's head.
3. Place the hands over the casualty's shoulder blades.
4. Rock forward to a vertical position to deflate the chest.
5. Rock back, at the same time lifting the elbows until resistance is felt: this expands the chest.

Repeat this cycle 12–14 times per minute, faster if possible for a child (with **less pressure** on the chest).

Although not as efficient as EAR, a sufficient exchange of air may take place for spontaneous breathing to be resumed.

6

Pregnancy and Emergency Childbirth

PREGNANCY

Pregnancy is a natural phenomenon, but certain things can go wrong which will require urgent attention. The most important of these are:
1. Antepartum haemorrhage (before delivery).
2. Postpartum haemorrhage (after delivery).
3. Eclamptic fits (toxaemia of pregnancy).
4. Miscarriage.

Antepartum haemorrhage

This shows as vaginal bleeding, usually originating behind the placenta (afterbirth) where it is attached to the wall of the uterus (womb); it may also occur from the cervix (neck of the womb) or elsewhere in the genital tract. All bleeding in pregnancy should be treated as serious. It is impossible to tell where the bleeding is coming from until the woman is examined by a doctor or midwife. Such bleeding may be accompanied by cramp-like abdominal pain, which may herald a miscarriage.

Reassurance is very important.

Treatment

1. Remove the patient to a quiet place. Note the number of pads or towels used and save them to enable blood loss to be estimated. Place her in a semi-recumbent position with her knees bent. This is usually the most comfortable position.
2. Allow the partner or a relative to comfort the patient.
3. **Do not** give anything to eat or drink, but the lips may be moistened with a damp tissue.
4. Call for an ambulance, stating that the patient is pregnant and bleeding.
5. Severe bleeding may require treatment for shock. Lay the patient down and elevate the legs.

Postpartum haemorrhage

This occurs following the birth of a baby. It may be due to bleeding from the uterus or following injury to the birth canal. Blood loss may have been continuing for some time without large apparent loss, but the sudden passage of large clots indicates significant bleeding.

Treatment

1. Note the number of pads used and save them.
2. Reassure the patient and allow her to assume the most comfortable position.
3. If the pulse is rapid and weak, lay the patient down and elevate her legs.
4. Call an ambulance immediately, and if possible contact the doctor or midwife who attended the birth.
5. **Do not** give anything by mouth.

Eclamptic fits

Sometimes the blood pressure becomes very high during pregnancy. Good antenatal care will usually pick up this complication early, before the woman becomes ill enough to develop fits. Occasionally, however, patients do not seek antenatal care, or will undertake long journeys away from medical supervision.

Symptoms and signs of eclampsia

Headache and disorientation may precede fitting or the fits may suddenly occur 'out of the blue'. Urgent medical aid is required to control the fits, and early delivery of the baby is required.

Treatment

1. Place the patient in the recovery position in a darkened room. Ensure an open airway.
2. Call an ambulance immediately, stating that the patient is pregnant and having fits.
3. Monitor respiration and pulse frequently.
4. Try not to restrain the patient, but place cushions or blankets under the head to prevent injury.

Miscarriage

A miscarriage (spontaneous abortion) may occur for many reasons. It is often nature's way of avoiding the birth of abnormal babies. It is most common at around the 8th to 16th week of pregnancy but can occur later. Twenty per cent of all pregnancies end in miscarriage.

Symptoms and signs

1. Vaginal bleeding. This may start as 'spotting', progressing to frank bleeding.
2. Cramp-like abdominal (labour) pains, which may become very distressing.
3. Expulsion of the fetus (baby) together with the placenta and membranes. The bleeding and pain may lead to shock. Not all of the products of conception may be passed. Everything which is passed must be retained, including all pads and towels used.

Treatment

1. Reassurance is vital. Keep calm.
2. Lay the patient down with her knees slightly bent, or in the most comfortable position. The woman may prefer to lie on her side.
3. Call an ambulance immediately, stating that a miscarriage is suspected.
4. Watch for signs of shock.

EMERGENCY CHILDBIRTH

Most births are normal deliveries, the mother and baby requiring very little assistance. In most cases labour is long enough to allow the patient to get to hospital, or in the case of a home confinement, to be attended by her doctor or midwife.

There are three stages of labour:
1. **First stage** – from the onset of regular contractions until the neck of the womb (cervix) is fully open (full dilatation).
2. **Second stage** – from the point of full dilatation until the baby is born.
3. **Third stage** – from the birth of the baby until the placenta (afterbirth) is delivered.

The first stage

Contractions usually begin slowly, sometimes accompanied by a low backache and a 'show' of bloodstained mucus from the vagina (this is the cervical mucus plug, which is expelled from the neck of the womb as it dilates). The contractions gradually increase in severity and backache may be severe. Eventually the membranes surrounding the baby will break (breaking of the waters) and amniotic fluid will be seen to escape from the vagina in quantities of up to a litre. Occasionally the membranes do not rupture until the cervix is fully dilated. The first stage of labour lasts several hours but is generally shorter for second and subsequent children.

Prolapsed cord

It may happen, in rare cases, that the umbilical cord protrudes from the cervix into the vagina following the escape of amniotic fluid. The baby receives all its oxygen via the cord and any interference with its blood supply (such as the baby's head pressing upon it) may be life-threatening for the baby.

When the membranes have ruptured, check to see that this has not occurred. If it has, the mother should be placed in the knee–elbow position (Fig. 6.1) to take pressure off the cord. Medical attention must be sought immediately. The ambulance service must be told that a prolapsed cord is suspected.

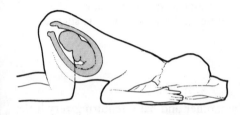

Fig. 6.1 The knee-elbow position.

Before touching the patient in the area of the birth canal, the hands must be thoroughly washed with soap and water and then again with antiseptic if available.

It is most important to respect the mother's privacy. She may be very embarrassed. If the first aider is male, he should ensure that he is chaperoned by a female (preferably a relative of the patient).

Reassurance is of paramount importance.

Remember that you are dealing with two patients, the mother *and* her baby.

It will rarely be necessary for a first aider to do any more than this, but if the second stage has begun he should proceed as follows.

The second stage

Keep calm. This reassures the mother that all is well. The second stage does not usually last much more than an hour and may be much shorter. If help is not already on its way, this must be summoned via the ambulance service. If possible, the hospital where the patient is booked for confinement, or her general practitioner, should be contacted by telephone as well. They will advise on further management until the ambulance arrives. If the situation is geographically remote and no help is available, the first aider must do what he or she can to help.

1. Allow the mother to lie on her side or semi-recumbent on a bed or couch. If out in the open, improvise a bed with coats or anoraks **in a sheltered spot**. Newspaper is relatively clean and can be used if no towels or sheets are available.

2. The mother should remove undergarments and tights or stockings. A towel or sheet affords some privacy but allows examination.

3. Contractions can be timed by asking the mother when the pains begin and end and by feeling the uterus through the abdominal wall. When they occur every two minutes or so, birth of the baby is imminent.

4. Improvise a mask by tying a handkerchief over the mouth and nose. Take off coats or jackets and roll up sleeves.

Do not allow anybody with a cold or cough to help. Wash hands thoroughly and scrub the nails with soap and water, preferably using a brush. Wash the hands again in antiseptic solution if available. If no washing facilities exist, avoid touching the baby or birth canal as much as possible.

5. Remember to keep the mother as warm and comfortable as possible. Continued reassurance is essential.

6. A crib may be improvised (if none is available) by lining a box or drawer with a blanket and then placing a clean sheet on top. Towels make very good, insulating cot blankets.

Delivery of the baby

If facilities allow, boil some scissors or a sharp knife for 15 minutes, as well as three pieces of string about 10 inches (25 cm) long. Boil some water and let it cool (in a **covered** pan) to cool down the instruments before use.

When the birth of the head is imminent, the mother will want to push. If she is on her back, tell her to put one foot on your hip (and the other on the hip of your assistant) and hold her head forward, chin on chest (the assistant's hand supporting her neck in the forward position). This allows the mother to make the maximum voluntary effort to expel the baby from the uterus. Ask the mother to take a large breath and push 'as though she were constipated' with each contraction, but to rest in between (allow her to take her feet down from your hip).

Cover the anus with a towel or pad.

As the head emerges, prevent it from 'rushing' out by gentle counter pressure with the hand. This will avoid sudden pressure changes which could cause bleeding into the baby's brain.

At this point check:

1. That the umbilical cord is not around the neck. If it is, gently lift it over the head.

2. That there is no membrane covering the baby's face.

3. That the baby's airway is not obstructed by blood or mucus. Wipe any away with a swab or clean handkerchief.

Do not pull on the baby's head.

The baby's head will rotate as the shoulders pass down the birth canal. Allow this to occur naturally, but maintain support to the head. As the shoulders are delivered, hold the baby firmly in a clean towel, lifting it onto the mother's abdomen. Newborn babies are wet and covered with a fatty substance. They are therefore very slippery.

Make sure that the baby's airway is clear and that he or she has started breathing. The baby will normally cry spontaneously, but if a breath is not taken within a moment or two, the baby can be stimulated by flicking its heels with a finger.

If this is to no avail, and there is deteriorating colour or marked pallor, commence artificial ventilation without further delay (mouth to baby's mouth and nose).

Feel for a pulse under the baby's left nipple and in the groin or neck.

If none is felt, commence full cardiopulmonary resuscitation.

The third stage

After the birth of the baby, there is an interval of a few minutes before the placenta is expelled. This may be assisted by massaging the mother's lower abdomen which encourages the uterus to contract. Watch the umbilical cord, which will lengthen as the placenta separates. The mother should be asked to push or cough at this point.

Do not pull on the cord.

It may break and allow the baby to bleed if the cord is still pulsating.

The third stage usually lasts ten to twenty minutes, but may take up to an hour. Provided there is no active bleeding, there is no danger if the placenta is not delivered before medical aid arrives.

Bleeding

Blood loss during delivery may be about a pint (600 ml or so), but is often much less. This is usually darkish red. Any quantity of bright red blood must be treated with suspicion and may indicate that either:

1. The uterus is not well contracted.

2. There has been an injury to the birth canal.

Loss greater than 600 ml constitutes 'postpartum haemorrhage'.

Treatment

1. Massage the lower abdomen.
2. Treat for shock.

Bleeding from the cord

The baby's blood volume is very small. If the cord is torn while it is still pulsating, the baby may suffer serious haemorrhage. If this occurs, take the pieces of previously boiled string and tie two ligatures around the baby's end of the cord about 5 cm (2 in) apart.

Cutting the cord

Normally the placenta should be left attached to the cord until medical help arrives. If the cord is very short, however, it may have to be cut. In order to do this safely, **wait until the cord has stopped pulsating** and then tie the three previously boiled pieces of string tightly around the cord at 10, 15 and 20 cm (4, 6 and 8 inches) from the baby's body. Cut the cord with the sterilized scissors (without touching the blades) between the second (15 cm) and third (20 cm) ligatures.

Do not discard the placenta.

The doctor or midwife will need to examine it to ensure that it is complete.
Wrap the cut end of the cord in a sterile dressing if available.

Abnormal births

Sometimes the baby is not born head first, or the head will not easily pass through the birth canal due to abnormal positioning inside the womb. There is little practical help the first aider can give in these situations unless the baby has passed through the birth canal buttocks first (breech delivery).

In all cases reassurance is invaluable.

Breech delivery

In a breech delivery, the buttocks are born first. The process of labour is similar to that for a normal delivery, except that the head is given much less time to traverse the birth canal. It is therefore subject to severe compression and rapid decompression. If this occurs too rapidly there is a danger of bleeding inside the baby's head.

1. As the baby's limbs are born, grasp them in a piece of clean material (to keep the baby warm and to afford a better grip).

2. Move the mother to the edge of the bed so that the baby may hang (gently supported) from the birth canal.

3. Exert gentle counter pressure against the mother's pushing as the shoulders become visible to prevent rapid expulsion of the head.

4. If, after 5 minutes, the head has not been born, firmly take the baby's feet and lift his body upward over the mother's abdomen so that the mouth and nose are visible. Clear the airway and gently support the baby until the rest of the head is born. Usually the baby is born face down but may be positioned as if looking over the mother's abdomen. In this case, the baby should be delivered rather more horizontally.

The baby should be kept wrapped in a towel at all times to prevent rapid heat loss from the wet skin.

When the baby is born, give it to the mother as soon as the airway has been cleared.

Part 2
Structure and Function

— 7

Cells, Tissues and Organs

Building blocks – the cells

All the cells in a person's body are derived from the fertilized egg, and although some develop into highly specialized structures, they all retain some features in common. A typical animal cell is shown in Fig. 7.1.

The cell is bounded by the **cell wall** which contains a jelly-like substance called **cytoplasm**. The cytoplasm itself contains structures concerned with energy production or the formation of secretions within the cell. Embedded in the cytoplasm is the **nucleus**, which contains the genetic material of the cell.

Tissues

Cells are collected together to form tissues. Cells become specialized (differentiated) to different degrees depending upon the tissue. For example,

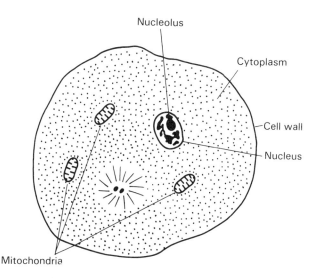

Fig. 7.1 A typical animal cell.

muscle and nerve cells are highly specialized, whereas cells of connective tissue (the 'supporting' tissue of the body) are less so. There are four basic types of tissue, the epithelium, connective and muscle tissue (see Chapter 12), and nerve tissue (see Chapter 10).

Epithelium may vary considerably in its appearance, but the same type of tissue covers the whole of the body surface including the bowel (which is properly regarded as outside the body – it is merely a channel through the body like a tunnel through a hillside). In the skin the cells become more flattened toward the surface and contain **keratin** (see below). Some epithelial surfaces are infolded to form **glands**. The skin merges with the membrane (mucous membrane) lining the bowel, nasal passages and genital passages to form one continuous layer.

The epithelial layer of the skin (Fig. 7.2) gives rise also to nail and hair. There are several layers, the outermost of which contains keratin which renders the skin waterproof. This is vital to prevent water loss from the body which readily occurs if a large area is damaged, as in a burn. The outer, cornified layer of skin consists of dead cells which are continually being shed. These are replaced by cells from the deeper layers.

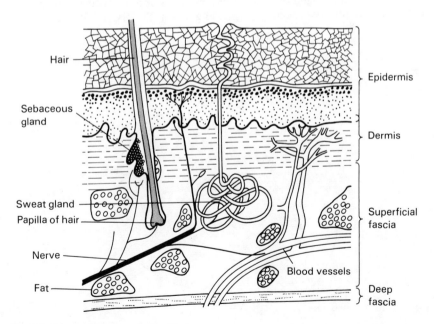

Fig. 7.2 Cross-section through the skin.

Functions of the skin

The skin has three main functions:
1. Protection from
   (a) trauma
   (b) excessive water loss
   (c) infection.
2. Temperature regulation (see Chapter 14).
3. Sense organs.
Many sense organs are sited in the skin, e.g. pain, temperature and 'touch' receptors. The skin has a rich nerve supply, especially in those areas an animal uses for assessing or manipulating an object (for example the finger pads in man).

Organs

Tissues are grouped together to form organs, which perform a particular function in the body. The stomach, for example, contains epithelial tissue, connective tissue, nerve and muscle.

— 8

The Respiratory System

The respiratory tract begins at the nostrils and lips and progressively includes the mouth and nasal cavities, the larynx, trachea, bronchi and lungs. The air is warmed and humidified in the oral and nasal cavities before it enters the larynx.

The larynx

This is a valve-like opening to the trachea. It closes during swallowing. The tracheal inlet is further protected by the **epiglottis**, a flap-like structure which folds over it. Halfway down the larynx lie the vocal cords (vocal folds). These produce the sound of speech, changes in pitch being effected by alterations in tension of the cords. If the nerve supply to the muscles controlling the vocal cords is cut, as may happen in injuries to the neck, the cords become paralysed and normal speech is lost.

The trachea and bronchi

These tubular structures convey air in and out of the lungs. The trachea is supported by cartilaginous hoops, as are the larger bronchi. The right and left main bronchi (Fig. 8.1(a)) divide into smaller and smaller branches.

The smallest branches are known as **bronchioles** (Fig. 8.1(b)). These lead to the air sacs where gas exchange between the air and the blood takes place (see below).

The lungs

There are two lungs, each divided into **lobes**, three on the right and two on the left. Each lung is covered with an epithelial membrane known as the **pleura**. It is this membrane which becomes inflamed in the condition known as pleurisy. The inside of the chest wall is also covered with a similar pleural membrane and the two layers lie close together, separated by only a thin film of fluid (Fig. 8.2). There is normally a subatmospheric (negative) pressure in this space, in other words a slight vacuum. It is this which draws air into the chest as it expands with the action of the intercostal muscles and diaphragm (see below).

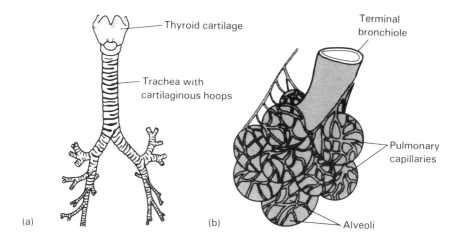

(a) (b)

Fig. 8.1(a) The trachea and main bronchi viewed from the front. (b) An air sac.

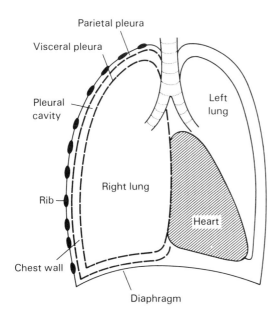

Fig. 8.2 The chest cavity showing the layers of pleura.

Any tearing of the pleura, such as a stab or bullet wound, will allow air at atmospheric pressure to enter the pleural cavity resulting in collapse of the lung on that side.

The **air sacs** themselves consist of many tiny 'pouches' called **alveoli**. Because of their large numbers there is a very large surface area available for exchange of oxygen into, and carbon dioxide out of, the blood.

An average adult breathes about one ton of oxygen each year! Room air contains 21% oxygen and virtually no carbon dioxide. About 16% oxygen and 4% carbon dioxide are found in expired air which, unlike room air, is saturated with water vapour. (Note that 16% oxygen in expired air is still sufficient to provide for the needs of a patient who is not breathing for himself. This is the principle underlying expired air or 'mouth to mouth' respiration.)

The mechanism of breathing

Expansion of the chest is brought about in two ways:
   (a)   the action of the diaphragm, and
   (b)   the action of the intercostal muscles.

The diaphragm is a muscular sheet separating the chest and abdominal cavities. Contraction of this muscle increases the depth of the chest cavity. The intercostal muscles lie between the ribs and move the ribs upwards and outwards when they contract, so increasing the diameter of the chest cavity (Fig. 8.3).

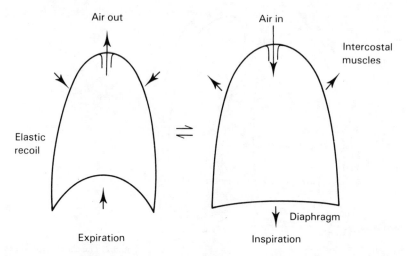

Fig. 8.3 The mechanism of respiration. The diaphragm is like an elastic sheet over the mouth of a jar.

Because these movements increase the volume of the chest cavity, the subatmospheric pressure (vacuum) within it increases, drawing air into the lungs (inspiration). Exhalation (expiration) is a **passive** process, except during coughing or sneezing when extra muscular force is applied.

Gas exchange

The combined thickness of the epithelial layers of the alveoli and the small blood vessels (capillaries) which form a close network around them, is about 0.5 mm. All gases entering or leaving the blood stream must traverse this membrane. In certain lung diseases the membrane becomes thickened, resulting in a barrier to the transfer of oxygen or carbon dioxide, particularly oxygen.

Oxygen transport

Oxygen which has entered the blood stream must be carried to all the tissues of the body. It is in the individual cells of the tissues that food energy (principally as glucose) is converted into carbon dioxide, water and energy. Some of the energy is released as heat but most is stored in special 'high energy' chemical compounds which are themselves used as fuel for specialized functions within the cell. Only a tiny fraction of the oxygen is carried in solution; most is combined loosely with the pigment **haemoglobin**, which gives blood its red colour. This raises the amount of oxygen carried per decilitre (100 ml) of blood from 0.3 ml (in simple solution) to 20 ml. Thus it is easy to see why anaemia (lack of haemoglobin) results in breathlessness!

The tissues of muscles and organs become more acid because of the breakdown products of metabolism, and there is more carbon dioxide than in the lungs. Here the oxygen dissociated from the haemoglobin passes into the tissue fluid and thence to the cells.

Carbon dioxide transport

Carbon dioxide combines loosely with proteins in the blood including haemoglobin, but it is also transported in simple solution and as bicarbonate.

The control of respiration

This is achieved by two mechanisms·
  (a)   nervous control, and
  (b)   chemical control.
The 'respiratory centre' in the brain is responsible for initiating the nervous impulses which ultimately bring about contraction of the respiratory muscles in a rhythmical fashion. Certain 'receptors' in the circulation and brain are

very sensitive to the acidity of the blood and the amount of carbon dioxide present. Normally the carbon dioxide content of the blood is controlled to within very narrow limits. Any increase results in greater respiratory effort in an attempt to eliminate the excess.

Cyanosis

When haemoglobin is oxygenated it is bright red in colour. Arterial blood is therefore usually bright red. In contrast, deoxygenated blood is darker. When the amount of deoxygenated blood exceeds 5 g per decilitre, a bluish colour appears in the skin. This is termed **cyanosis**. It may not be seen when the amount of haemoglobin present is much less than normal as in severe anaemia.

Cyanosis, if seen in the lips or mouth, usually indicates a respiratory or circulatory disorder. It is also commonly seen in the fingers or ear lobes and may then be the result of cold interfering with the blood supply to the part, or compression of an artery, for example by tight clothing, or even just an unconscious person lying upon a limb.

9

The Heart and Circulation

The mammalian heart, including that of man, has evolved from a simple tubular structure. In the embryo a simple tubular heart becomes folded upon itself resulting in a four chambered heart (Fig. 9.1).

The heart is enclosed in a tough membrane (the pericardium) containing a thin layer of fluid. The heart is composed almost entirely of muscle and is essentially a pump, or more correctly two pumps. These are termed the right and left heart respectively. Each consists of two chambers, an **atrium** and a **ventricle** (Fig. 9.2).

The right and left heart, however, beat almost synchronously. The right heart receives **deoxygenated** blood from the body and pumps it to the lungs. The left heart receives **oxygenated** blood from the lungs and pumps it around the rest of the body. Vessels taking blood away from the heart are called **arteries**, those returning blood to it **veins**. The main artery leaving the heart is the **aorta**. It divides successively into smaller vessels (Fig. 9.3).

The **coronary arteries**, which supply the heart muscle itself with blood, also arise from the aorta, but unlike the other arteries most of the flow in them occurs in the relaxation phase, when the heart is filling.

Electrical conduction in the heart

Heart muscle is arranged as a network, each fibre of which has the capacity to contract rhythmically. In addition to this network, the presence of special **conducting tissue** results in these muscle fibres producing coordinated contraction. There is a natural pacemaker in the normal heart, situated high up in the wall of the right atrium (sinoatrial node) (Fig. 9.1). Impulses spread from there through the conducting tissue to the ventricles. Since all of the conducting tissue will respond to a wave of stimulation spreading down from the pacemaker, the heart rate is controlled (60–80 beats per minute in the resting adult). Babies have a much faster heart rate, up to 140 beats per minute.

Blood pressure

Blood pressure can most easily be visualized by recalling the history of its measurement. In the 17th century, the Reverend Stephen Hales inserted a tube into an artery of a horse and noted that the column of blood rose to an

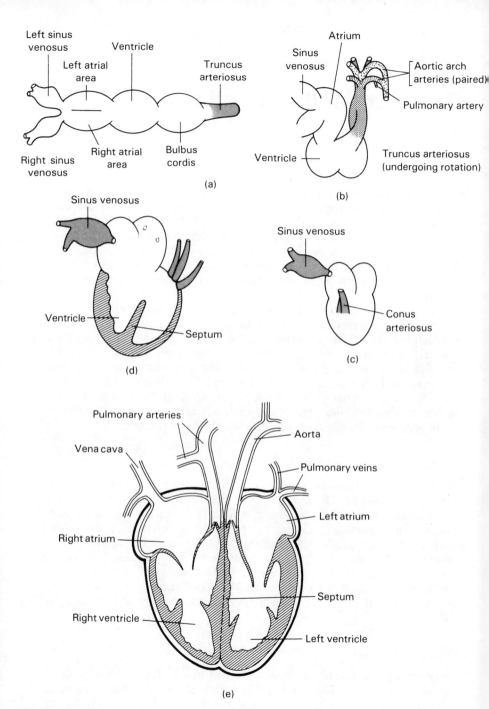

Fig. 9.1 Development of the heart.

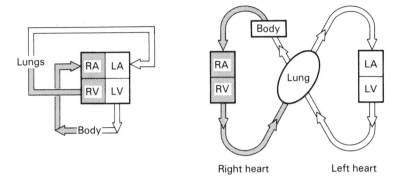

Fig. 9.2 The heart is made up of two pumps.

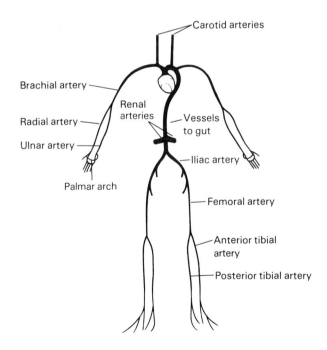

Fig. 9.3 The major arteries.

appreciable height above the level of the artery. The height of this column of blood above the level of the artery is the blood pressure (measured in inches or centimetres of blood).

Blood pressure is now commonly referred to as the height of a column of mercury this pressure would support. It is on average 120 mm (4.7 in) of mercury. The blood pressure is lower in children.

It is not easy to measure the amount of blood pumped by the heart with each beat or in each minute, but the blood pressure which is thereby generated can be easily measured. It gives important information about the state of the heart and circulation. A certain amount of pressure is required to drive the blood around the body. If the pressure is too high, organs may be damaged. If it is too low, the tissues may not be adequately oxygenated or their waste products cleared.

The pressure referred to so far is that generated by the left side of the heart. The pulmonary circulation serving the lungs is also maintained by a blood pressure generated by the right side of the heart. This is normally much lower than the blood pressure in the rest of the body.

Response to exercise

The blood flow to muscle increases enormously during vigorous exercise in response to the increased demand for oxygen, which may be as much as 200% of the resting value. The heart rate may treble but the blood pressure rises only very little. This is due to blood vessels in the muscle 'opening up' (vasodilation) to accommodate the extra blood flow.

Postural changes

When body position is altered, for example on rising from a bed, blood collects in the veins of the legs. This results in compensatory reflexes coming into play causing the small blood vessels in the lower limbs to tighten up, preventing a fall in blood pressure and maintaining adequate return of blood to the heart and thence to the brain. On a warm day, or after a hot bath, insufficient constriction of the vessels may occur with a consequent fall in blood pressure. The person then feels faint. Under normal circumstances the intermittent contraction of the leg muscles helps to pump blood through the veins ('muscle pump'). When these muscles are inactive, such as when soldiers stand to attention for long periods, a similar pooling effect occurs and fainting may ensue.

Blood

The composition of blood

Blood may be regarded as one of the body's connective tissues. It is made up of water, proteins, simple and complex chemicals in solution and various

blood cells. The fluid portion is called **plasma**. It contains proteins responsible for the clotting of blood. When clotting has occurred, i.e. when the blood has separated into its component parts, the fluid remaining is termed **serum**.

Blood cells

There are two main types, **red cells** and **white cells**. They are formed in the bone marrow.

Red cells are doughnut shaped with a depression in the centre (Fig. 9.4). They have no nuclei but contain large amounts of the red pigment haemoglobin. Haemoglobin is responsible for nearly all the oxygen carrying capacity of the blood. Red cells have a life span of about 120 days; after that time they are removed by the spleen.

White cells possess nuclei and are much larger than the red cells. There are several types, and all are concerned with the body's defence mechanisms. Some actively 'scavenge' cell debris and bacteria, which they engulf. Others are concerned with recognition of substances foreign to the body, and with the production of antibodies.

(a)

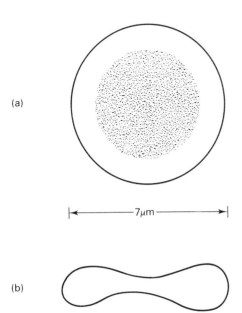

├─────7μm─────┤

(b)

Fig. 9.4 The red cell: (a) seen from above; (b) cross-section.

Platelets

These are not true cells, but consist of pieces of protoplasm of the large white cells from which they are derived. They are concerned with the clotting of blood.

The composition of the blood is very precisely controlled by the body.

Functions of the blood:

1. Oxygen transport.
2. Carbon dioxide transport.
3. Energy transport.
4. Chemical transport.
5. Protection against infection.
6. Healing processes (blood clotting and 'organization' into scar tissue).

The lymph

Fluid which leaves the circulation to become tissue fluid eventually returns via the **lymphatic system**, a system of vessels similar to blood vessels which eventually enter the venous system. Along the length of these vessels are lymph **nodes** ('glands') containing white cells which form part of the immune system.

The clotting of blood

When tissue is damaged and blood vessels are cut, chemical substances are released – from the tissues and from the circulating platelets – which cause certain proteins (e.g. fibrinogen) in the blood to link together in chains. These chains form a 'meshwork' which traps blood cells, thus plugging the wound. Eventually the clot shrinks and dries out forming a waterproof covering to the wound. As the wound heals, the clot 'organizes' into new tissue.

— 10

The Nervous System and Sense Organs

THE NERVOUS SYSTEM

The nervous system is the main coordinating mechanism of the body. It consists of the central and autonomic nervous systems. The central nervous system comprises the brain, from which the cranial nerves pass, and the spinal cord, from which the spinal nerves form peripheral nerves. The autonomic nervous system controls the involuntary actions of the body.

Nerve tissue

The nervous system is made up of the special nerve cells and the nerve fibres which emerge from them (Fig. 10.1). Nerve cells are located in the brain and spinal cord, and together form the grey matter of the nervous system. Each cell has a long projection, called the fibre or **axon**, and a number of fine interlacing branches known as **dendrites**. These nerve fibres vary in length according to the distance which they have to travel. Fibres from the sole of the feet carrying impulses to the spinal cord through the sciatic nerve are the longest fibres in the body.

The dendrites pick up impulses and carry them into the cell while the axon carries the impulse **from** the cell. The axon ends by dividing into a number of branches which communicate either with the dendrites of another cell or with the special structures of a tissue such as muscle.

Nerve fibres can only carry messages in one direction. Those nerves which convey sensation to the brain and spinal cord are called sensory nerves, while those which convey impulses of movement to the muscles are called motor fibres. Sensory nerves consist of bundles of sensory fibres grouped together, and motor nerves are bundles of motor fibres. Mixed nerves (the most common type) are nerves in which both sensory and motor nerve fibres can be found.

Within the central nervous system (the brain and spinal cord) the nerve fibres are grouped together to form the white matter. Grey matter, which is the collection of nerve cells, is found in the brain and spinal cord but not in peripheral nerves. Grey matter is also found in the small isolated masses of nerve cells, the ganglia, which are found close to the spinal cord in the autonomic nervous system.

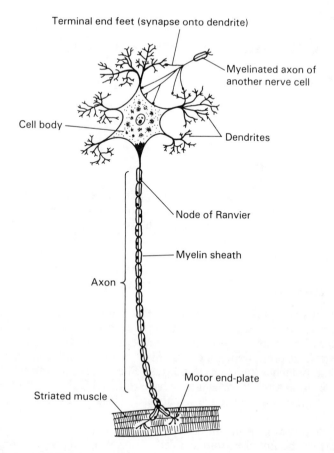

Terminal end feet (synapse onto dendrite)

Myelinated axon of another nerve cell

Cell body

Dendrites

Node of Ranvier

Myelin sheath

Axon

Motor end-plate

Striated muscle

Fig. 10.1 A nerve cell (neuron).

The central nervous system

The central nervous system controls all the muscles of the head, trunk and limbs. It is the seat of all sensation, of the intellect, emotions, reason and will-power (Fig. 10.2).

The brain

The brain is a large, delicate organ which almost fills the cavity of the skull. It weighs about 1.5 kg. Its relatively large size compared to the total weight of the body is one of the main differences between man and the animals.

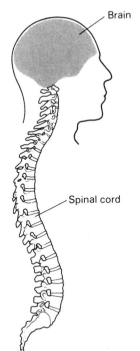

Brain

Spinal cord

Fig. 10.2 Side view of the nervous system.

There are four main parts of the brain:
(a) the cerebrum,
(b) the cerebellum,
(c) the pons, and
(d) the medulla oblongata.

The cerebrum forms the greater part of the human brain. It is divided into two large hemispheres, right and left, each of which controls the opposite side of the body. A message from the left cerebral hemisphere will pass to the right side of the body and vice versa.

The cerebrum consists of grey matter on the surface and white matter in the centre. The surface is thrown into a number of ridges called convolutions, which greatly increase the brain capacity. Function has been localized to several of these convolutions (as shown in Fig. 10.3).

The cerebellum also consists of two hemispheres with grey matter on the surface and white matter in the centre; its surface is thrown into convolutions finer than those of the cerebrum. It lies below and behind the cerebrum and has the important function of controlling the coordination of muscles; acting with the cerebrum it produces skilled, steady movement and controls posture.

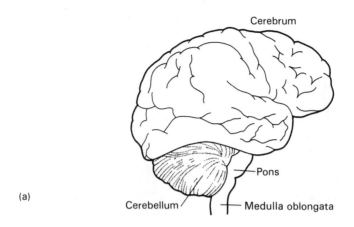

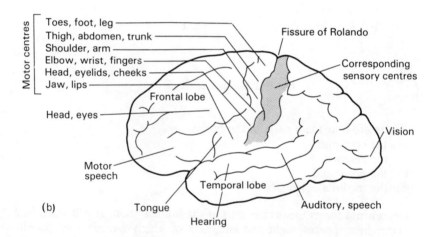

Fig. 10.3 Side view of the brain: (a) showing main structures; (b) showing various centres.

The pons (which together with the medulla forms the brainstem) is a bridge of nerve fibres which join together the various parts of the brain, linking the two hemispheres of the cerebellum and joining the cerebrum above to the medulla below.

The medulla oblongata joins the brain to the spinal cord, being continuous with the pons above and the cord below. It consists of motor fibres running down from the brain to the cord, and sensory fibres running up from the cord to the brain. Both the motor and sensory fibres cross in the medulla, causing the right side of the brain to control the left side of the body.

Within the medulla are the vital centres which control the essential activities of life, i.e. respiration and circulation; they are the respiratory, cardiac and vasomotor centres. If the vital centres are damaged and cease to function death will occur. On the other hand, if only the higher centres of the brain cease to function, following damage in a head injury, life may continue with the heart and the lungs still functioning. This is called 'brain death'.

The spinal cord

This is a cylinder of nerve tissue about 18 in long, running through the spinal canal. It joins the medulla oblongata above, and ends at the lower level of the first lumbar vertebra, continuing as a bunch of nerves called the cauda equina. These nerves go to the pelvis and to the lower limbs.

Structure of the spinal cord. As seen in the diagram of a cross-section of the spinal cord (Fig. 10.4) the spinal cord consists of white matter on the surface with grey matter in the centre. The white matter consists of:
1. Motor fibres bringing messages (impulses) from the motor centres of the brain to the motor cells of the anterior horn of the cord.

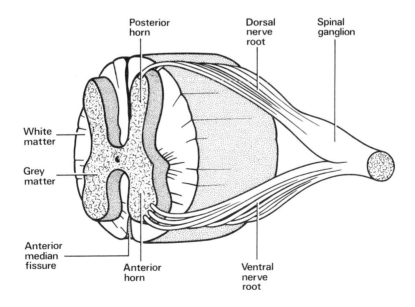

Fig. 10.4 Cross-section of the spinal cord.

2. Sensory fibres carrying messages from the sensory cells of the spinal cord to the sensory cells of the brain.

The grey matter consists of both motor and sensory cells and forms an H-shape. The motor cells lie in the anterior horn and give off the motor fibres which run out to the muscles, forming the motor fibres of the spinal nerves. Messages from the motor centres of the brain travel down the spinal cord to these motor nerve cells and are then relayed to other cells in the anterior horn and thence to the various muscles. The sensory fibres of the spinal nerves bring impulses from the tissues and skin. These impulses are picked up in the sensory cells in the posterior horns. Some relay as a reflex, others are passed on to the brain running up the sensory fibres in the spinal cord. In the brain we now recognize them as sensations of pain, temperature, cold etc. and can relate them to a specific part of the body.

The cranial nerves

The cranial nerves come from the brain and supply various organs of the head and neck. There are 12 pairs, which may be **motor, sensory,** or **mixed.**

The motor cranial nerves include the important facial nerves to the muscles of expression of the face, the fine nerves which supply the muscles of the eye, and the hypoglossal nerve to the tongue.

Sensory cranial nerves are the optic nerves (sight), the auditory nerves (hearing), and the olfactory nerves (smell).

Mixed cranial nerves contain both motor and sensory fibres. The trigeminal or 5th cranial nerve supplies muscles of mastication, which move the jaw, and also important fibres carrying sensations from the face and teeth.

The vagus, or 10th cranial nerve, is an important mixed cranial nerve which supplies all the internal organs of the chest and upper part of the gut. It forms an important part of the autonomic nervous system (see Fig. 10.5).

The spinal nerves

31 pairs of spinal nerves come from the spinal cord. They supply the muscles of the trunk and limbs with motor fibres which produce movement, and to a lesser extent provide the muscles, bones and joints with sensory fibres, giving them sensation; they also supply the skin richly with sensory fibres.

The spinal nerves are therefore mixed, carrying both motor fibres and sensory fibres. The motor fibres pass from the motor cell in the anterior horn of grey matter to the muscles, whilst the sensory fibres arise in the specialized nerve endings of the skin and pass to the sensory cells in the posterior horn of the grey matter of the cord (see Fig. 10.4).

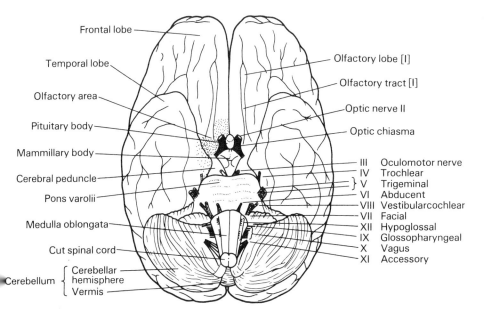

Fig. 10.5 Cranial nerves emerging from base of brain.

The meninges

The brain and spinal cord are covered by three membranes called the meninges. The outer coat is a tough fibrous sheath which lines the cranium and spinal canal and is called the dura mater. The middle coat, called the arachnoid, is a delicate membrane which loosely envelopes brain and spinal cord (see Fig. 10.6).

The inner coat, the pia mater, is a very thin membrane rich in blood vessels and adherent to the surface of the brain, dipping into all its convolutions. Between the pia and arachnoid maters lies the cerebrospinal fluid, which is a clear watery fluid that serves as a waterbed or cushion to protect the brain and cord. It also nourishes the brain cells, and is constantly formed and drained away into the circulation.

Autonomic nervous system

The autonomic system controls the involuntary muscles of the various internal organs such as the stomach and intestines, the bladder, the heart and the tiny muscles controlling the diameter of the blood vessels (Fig. 10.7). A person is not conscious of the normal activities of the autonomic system, nor is he able to control them; for example, the contraction of the bowel is not

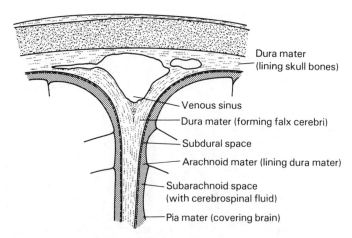

Fig. 10.6 Cross section of skull, showing brain, dura, arachnoid and pia mater.

normally felt by the individual. However, following interference with the blood supply (ischaemia), distension or abnormal contractions (colic) of the bowel, i.e. abnormal sensations, will be felt. These are related to the surface of the body; as another example, the pain occurring after a coronary thrombosis will be felt in the chest and along the left arm.

SENSE ORGANS

There are many different types of structure in the body concerned with our appreciation of our surroundings. Some, such as the eye and ear, are obvious, but others such as those concerned with appreciation of pain and touch are much less so.

Touch, pain and pressure

In the skin especially, but also in other tissues, are receptors which are sensitive to touch, temperature, pressure and pain. Pain and temperature sensations are closely linked, and their nerve fibres travel in the same portion of the spinal cord. It is possible that different stimuli as applied to a single type of receptor may produce different sensations.

Position sense

There are receptors situated in the muscles, joints and tendons which help an animal to appreciate its position in space. This is also assisted by the semicircular canals (see below).

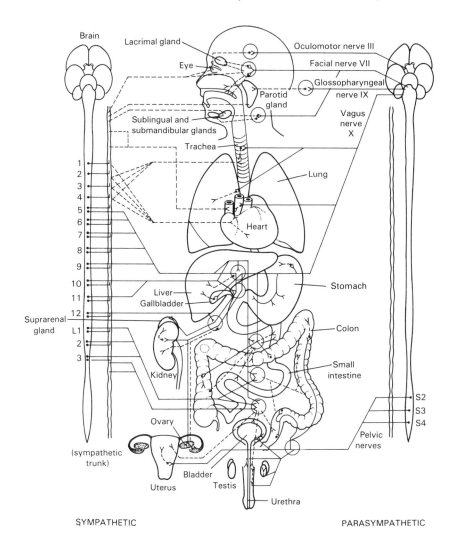

Fig. 10.7 Autonomic nervous system.

Other receptors

In the circulatory system are chemical receptors involved with the control of respiration, and pressure-sensitive receptors concerned with the control of blood pressure.

Specialized sense organs

We shall discuss briefly the eye, the sense of smell, the ear and the sense of balance.

The eye

The eyeball is roughly spherical and is about 2.5 cm (1 in) in diameter. It has two compartments, separated by the **lens** and its associated muscles. The chamber in front of the lens is filled with a watery fluid, **the aqueous humour**, while the compartment behind is filled with a jelly-like fluid, **the vitreous humour**. The front of the eye is covered by the **conjunctiva**. It blends with the skin of the eyelid and is only one cell thick over the **cornea** or transparent part of the eye (Fig. 10.8).

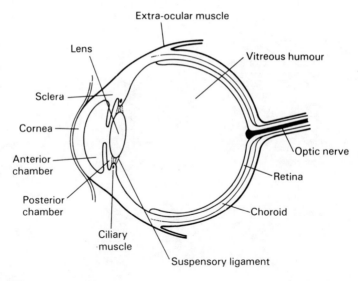

Fig. 10.8 The globe of the eye.

The innermost coat of the eyeball is the **retina**, which contains the light sensitive elements, pigment cells and the fibres of the optic nerve. The retina occasionally becomes detached from the globe, which causes vision to be seriously affected.

The **lacrimal gland** is situated in the upper part of the bony eye socket (the orbit). It produces tears which keep the sensitive cornea clean and moist. There are six muscles within the orbit which move the eyeball in all directions. If the muscles of the two eyes do not work together properly, a squint develops (strabismus).

The sense of smell

This is conveyed from the chemical receptors in the nose by many hundreds of **olfactory nerves,** passing upwards to the olfactory bulb of the brain. The sense of smell is poorly developed in humans by comparison with other mammals, such as the dog. The sense of taste is closely linked with that of smell, and is thus often affected when a person has a cold. Fractures of the base of the skull may lead to damage to the olfactory nerves, with consequent loss of the sense of smell.

The ear

The senses of hearing and balance are anatomically contained within the ear.

The external ear consists of the pinna (the 'ear') and the external ear canal. The external ear is separated from the middle ear cavity by the **tympanic membrane** or 'eardrum' (Fig. 10.9).

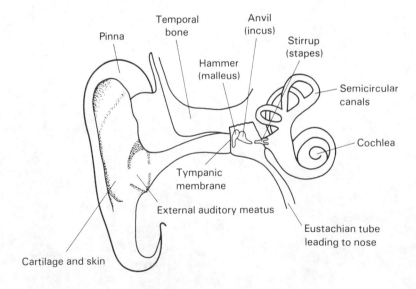

Fig. 10.9 The ear.

The middle ear is contained within the bone of the base of the skull. It contains three small bones called the 'hammer', 'anvil' and 'stirrup' because of their shapes. Collectively they are known as the **ossicles** and serve to amplify the sound waves (vibrations) reaching the eardrum. The footplate of the stirrup rests on the structure called the **oval window**. It transmits the sound waves to the fluid-filled, shell-like **cochlea** which contains the sensory cells and forms part of the inner ear.

The inner ear is made up of the structures containing the sense organs of hearing (the cochlea) and balance (the labyrinth). The labyrinth consists in part of three semicircular canals which are filled with fluid. They are situated at right angles to each other. Movement in any direction can be detected by sensory cells within the canals, as the fluid moves relative to the canals.

— 11

The Skeleton

The human skeleton gives form and a framework to the body. It protects the vital organs such as the brain, heart and lungs, and consists of 206 bones, 86 of which are paired and 34 single. Bones are generally classified as being long, short, flat or irregular.

Long bones

The central bones of the limbs form a system of levers. They consist of a cylinder of compact bone with a medullary cavity containing marrow and blood vessels. The bone ends are cancellous or 'spongy' bone with a thin outer shell of compact bone. Examples of long bones are the femur, radius, and metacarpals (Fig. 11.1).

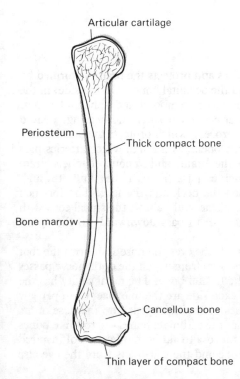

Articular cartilage

Periosteum

Thick compact bone

Bone marrow

Cancellous bone

Thin layer of compact bone

Fig. 11.1 Longitudinal section through a long bone.

Short bones

Short bones are spongy, cancellous bone covered by a thin layer of compact bone. The bones of the carpus or wrist are examples of short bones.

Flat bones

Flat bones consist of two layers of compact bone with spongy, cancellous bone sandwiched between. This type of bone is found in the skull.

Irregular bones

Irregular bones have an outer layer of compact bone with a varying amount of spongy bone within. Their shape varies according to their site and function. Some of those in the skull, the pneumatic bones, have air spaces which give lightness to the structure.

The skeleton (Fig. 11.2) can be divided generally into two parts, the **axial skeleton**, consisting of the skull and vertebral column, and the **appendicular skeleton**, consisting of the upper and lower limbs and the pelvic and shoulder girdles.

THE AXIAL SKELETON

The skull

The cranium (Fig. 11.3) which encloses and protects the brain, is formed by the large frontal, the two parietal and the occipital bones. On the side, in the temporal fossa, are the flat portions of the temporal and sphenoid bones. Within the temporal bone is the inner ear, for balance and hearing. Behind the opening to the ear is the mastoid process, which protects the facial nerve. The strong base of the skull has many openings through which arteries pass into the skull, to supply blood to the brain, and venous channels drain outwards. The important cranial nerves pass through the skull, through special openings and canals, to reach the neck and the face. The foramen magnum, a large opening in the base of the skull, allows the spinal cord with its meningeal coverings (see Chapter 10) to pass downwards to the spinal canal.

The facial part of the skull surrounds the eyes and nose and forms the roof of the mouth. The two orbits (eye sockets) from which the optic nerve passes backwards to the brain, lie below the frontal bone. The nasal cavity has the small nasal bone anteriorly, and on each side are the maxillae, or upper jaw bones, which contain large air sinuses. The sinus opens into the nose on its lateral side. The inside of the nose has the turbinate bones – scroll-like bones which increase the area of the nasal mucosa to aid humidification of inspired air. Two sinuses from the frontal bone and the tear ducts from the eye also

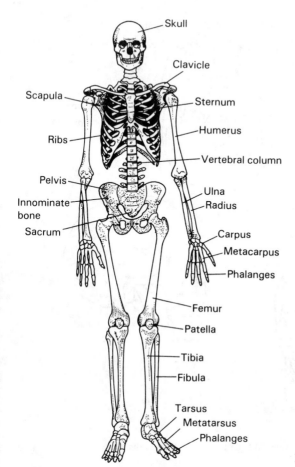

Fig. 11.2 The skeleton.

open into the nasal cavity. The cheek bone (the zygomatic bone) lies on the outer side of the maxilla and forms the outer wall of the orbits. The lower edge of the maxilla (the alveolar margin) contains the teeth. The horizontal portions of the maxillae unite with the palatine bone to form the hard palate, the roof of the mouth. The jaw bone (the mandible) consists of a strong horizontal portion which contains teeth and to which the tongue is attached. A vertical portion has a condyle at the top, which articulates with the base of the skull.

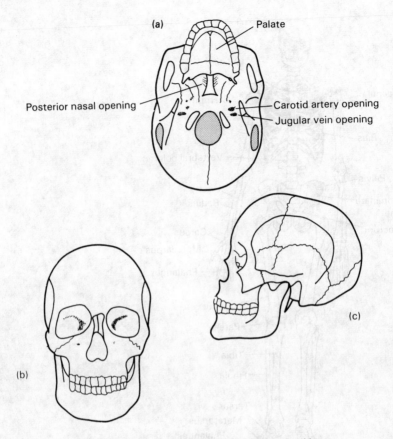

Fig. 11.3 The skull (a) from below; (b) from the front; (c) from the side.

The vertebral column

Thirty-three vertebrae, irregular bones joined by strong intervertebral discs, support the trunk and give protection to the spinal cord (see Figs. 11.4 and 11.5). Each vertebra has a body of cancellous bone covered by compact bone, and within this is bone marrow which forms red cells. Many large veins pass in and out.

The vertebral arch surrounds and protects the spinal cord and its meningeal linings. Transverse processes jut out from this arch, to which

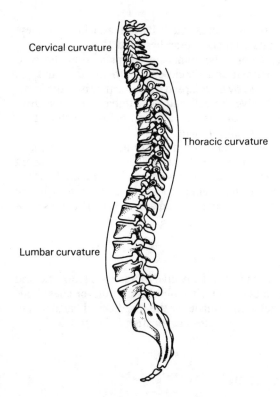

Cervical curvature

Thoracic curvature

Lumbar curvature

Fig. 11.4 The spine or vertebral column.

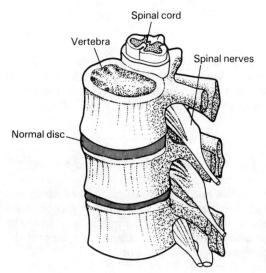

Spinal cord

Vertebra

Spinal nerves

Normal disc

Fig. 11.5 Typical vertebrae including the vertebral disc.

muscles are attached, and in the thorax the ribs are attached to these processes. Small synovial joints connect the arches, and the intervertebral discs connect the vertebral bodies. The spinal nerves pass from the cord through the intervertebral foramen and lie close to both the disc and the joints. There they may be irritated by a prolapsed disc or arthritis in the joint.

There are seven cervical, twelve thoracic and five lumbar vertebrae. Five sacral vertebrae are fused together to form the sacrum, below which lie four vestigial coccygeal vertebrae, the tail remnant.

The several curves in the vertebral column add to its elasticity and give increased resistance to the transmitted weight, as well as allowing movement in different directions. The sacrum articulates with two innominate bones to form the strong pelvic girdle. Strong ligaments connect these bones. In the female during pregnancy, these soften to allow expansion for the baby's head to be born.

Thoracic cage

Twelve ribs on each side are attached to the twelve thoracic vertebrae behind (see Fig. 11.6). In front the upper seven ribs join the sternum or chest bone by costal cartilages. The costal arch is made by the fused costal cartilages of the next three ribs. The 11th and 12th ribs are 'floating' ribs, to which only muscles are attached.

THE APPENDICULAR SKELETON

The upper limb

The clavicle

The collar bone (Fig. 11.7) with two gentle curves braces the shoulders back. Strong ligaments connect it to the sternum on the medial side and to the coracoid process of the scapula on the lateral side. The weight of the arm is carried by this bone and all movements of the arm rotate around it.

The scapula

This is a triangular flat bone (Fig. 11.8) with a dorsal spine and a strong bar of bone which forms the lateral border. Many muscles hold the humerus in the shoulder joint, and large muscles run from the trunk to the scapula and rotate it around the chest. The shoulder joint has the shallow glenoid fossa with a fibrocartilaginous ring, to which the joint capsule is attached. The coracoid process projects forwards; it has a strong ligament to support the weight of the arm and muscles pass from it to the arm.

The clavicle and scapula together form the pectoral (shoulder) girdle.

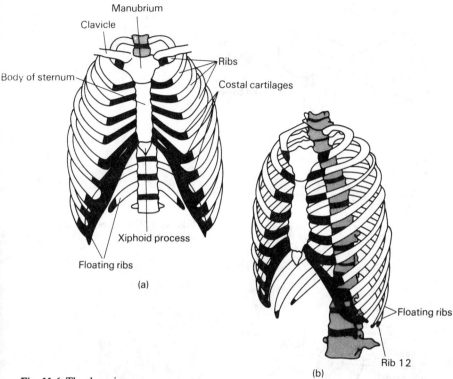

Fig. 11.6 The thoracic cage.

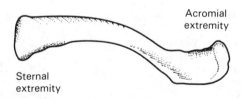

Fig. 11.7 The clavicle. Note: the term 'extremity' when applied to a bone means 'end'.

The humerus

The humerus (Fig. 11.9) is a long bone with many prominent markings on it which are the attachment points of strong muscles. The rounded head articulates with the glenoid fossa of the scapula. The scapular muscles are attached to the two tuberosities and hold it closely during movement. The

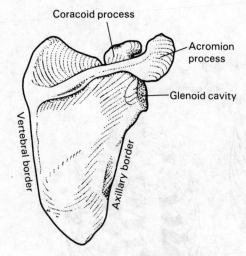

Fig. 11.8 The scapula (seen from behind).

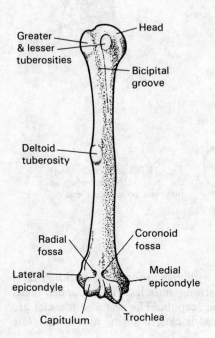

Fig. 11.9 The humerus.

'surgical neck' lies just below the head and is commonly fractured. The nerve to the deltoid muscle passes around the surgical neck and this is often injured when the shoulder is dislocated. The shaft, which is strong and tubular, has many muscular markings. The trochlea, on the lower end of the humerus, articulates with the upper end of the ulna, and lateral to the trochlea lies the spherical capitulum on which the head of the radius can rotate.

The ulna

The expanded upper end of the ulna (Fig. 11.10) has a fossa which forms a hinge joint with the humerus. The prominent olecranon process forms the point of the elbow and has the strong triceps muscle attached, which straightens the elbow. The shaft has many muscular markings and on the lateral side a strong membrane connects it to the radius. The lower end has a small styloid process with a triangular cartilage, which holds it to the radius.

The radius

The head or upper end of the radius has a concavity on the top and a smooth circumference where it rotates on the ulna. The bicipital tuberosity receives

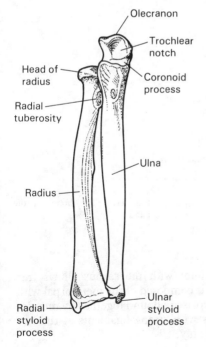

Fig. 11.10 The radius and ulna.

the tendon of the strong biceps muscle. The medial border of the shaft has the interosseous membrane attached to it; this transmits force from the hand and wrist, as well as giving a large surface for muscle attachments. The lower portion is grooved by tendons running over the bone. The lower smooth surface articulates with the wrist bones. The prominent styloid process has a strong ligament attached to it. On the medial side is a smooth area to receive the head of the ulna.

The wrist and hand

The eight small bones of the wrist or carpus (Fig. 11.11) articulate in two rows of four bones. They are small bones with several ligaments, which allow a larger composite movement. The thumb has a short, stumpy metacarpal

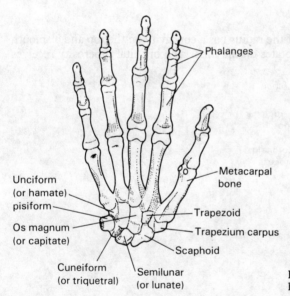

Phalanges

Unciform
(or hamate)
pisiform

Os magnum
(or capitate)

Cuneiform
(or triquetral)

Semilunar
(or lunate)

Scaphoid

Trapezium carpus

Trapezoid

Metacarpal
bone

Fig. 11.11 The bones of the hand.

with two phalanges; a separate saddle joint with the carpus allows free movement. Each of the other four fingers is composed of the metacarpal with three phalanges. These other four metacarpals are bound together by muscles and ligaments. The fingers have capsules with strong ligaments at the two joints to allow free flexion and extension only.

The lower limb

The pelvis

The two innominate bones articulate with the sacrum (Fig. 11.12) by a flat synovial joint with strong interosseous ligaments. Anteriorly, the pubic bones are attached at the symphysis. The upper parts of these bones form a shallow bowl, part of the abdominal cavity. The true pelvis lies between the sacrum and the inner aspects of the ischium and pubic bones. On the inner aspect are attached the muscles of the floor of the pelvis, the levatores ani, which support the bladder, uterus and rectum. The large sciatic notch transmits the sciatic nerve as well as other nerves, arteries and a large muscle. The back of the ilium has muscular markings for the gluteal muscles, which balance the body on the thigh bone. On the lateral aspect of the pubis, the deep acetabulum receives the femoral head. Below this is the strong ischial tuberosity on which we sit, and to which are attached the hamstring muscles. Marked sexual differences may be seen in the pelvic bones.

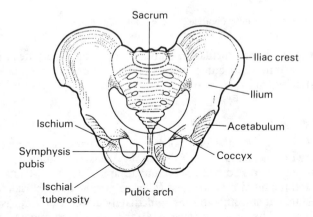

Fig. 11.12 The pelvis.

The femur

The femur (Fig. 11.13) is a long, strong bone with a prominent globular head and a long neck at an angle to the shaft. The greater and lesser trochanters form attachments for the muscles around the hip joint. On the posterior aspect of the shaft are strong muscle markings for the buttock muscles and the linea aspera for thigh muscle attachments. The lower femur has two large condyles: these are shaped to articulate inferiorly with the upper surface of the

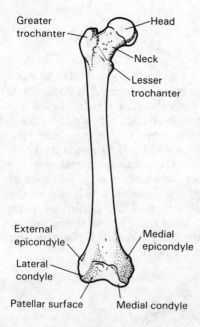

Greater
trochanter

Head

Neck

Lesser
trochanter

External
epicondyle

Medial
epicondyle

Lateral
condyle

Patellar surface

Medial condyle

Fig. 11.13 The femur.

tibia and the semilunar cartilages, and anteriorly with the patella (see Fig. 12.4). On the inner and outer aspects of these condyles are markings for ligament attachments.

The tibia

The tibia (Fig. 11.14) is a long bone with an expanded upper end which articulates with the femur. Its upper surface has two smooth areas. The central portion is raised with attachment areas for the strong cruciate ligaments and the meniscal cartilages. The shaft of the bone is triangular, and its medial side, flat and smooth, lies immediately under the skin, easily felt as the shin bone. The lower surface with the prominent medial malleolus articulates with the upper surface of the talus.

The fibula

The fibula is a thin, twisted bone with many surfaces for the attachment of muscles. The prominent head articulates with the tibia. A large nerve passes close to the neck at the upper end and is easily damaged by pressure. The expanded lower portion, the lateral malleolus, is joined to the tibia by a strong interosseous ligament. The lateral ligament attaches the fibula to the bones of the foot and is often sprained.

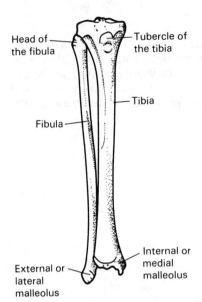

Head of the fibula

Tubercle of the tibia

Tibia

Fibula

Internal or medial malleolus

External or lateral malleolus

Fig. 11.14 The bones of the leg (tibia and fibula).

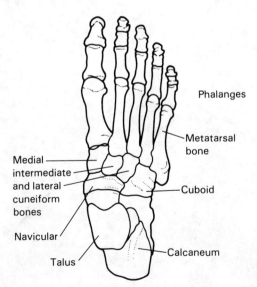

Phalanges

Metatarsal bone

Medial intermediate and lateral cuneiform bones

Cuboid

Navicular

Talus

Calcaneum

Fig. 11.15 The bones of the foot.

The foot

The foot (Fig. 11.15) has seven tarsal bones: the talus, os calcis, navicular, cuboid and three cuneiform bones. These are small bones which glide over each other for short distances. The five metatarsals have the phalanges attached to them. The great toe has two phalanges whilst the others have three. They form a flexible platform with longitudinal and transverse arches which adjust to weight and movement.

12

Joints and the Muscular System

Joints

A joint or articulation is formed by the meeting of two or more bones.
These joints may be:
1. Immovable joints, such as the sutures between the bones of the skull (Fig. 12.1).
2. Slightly movable joints, the symphyses, as in the pelvis (Fig. 12.2).
3. Freely movable joints, mostly synovial (Figs. 12.3 and 12.4).

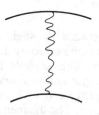

Fig. 12.1 Immovable joint (skull).

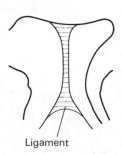

Ligament

Fig. 12.2 Slightly movable joint (symphysis pubis – front of pelvis).

The **freely movable,** or synovial joints, are the ones most frequently injured and it is important to learn more about their structure. The other two types of joints are dealt with in Chapters 20 and 25 respectively.

The two ends of the bone taking part in the joint or articulation are expanded cancellous bone covered by a thin layer of hard, compact bone. Over the joint surface, the articular end of the bone, is a layer of cartilage which is smooth and polished and enables the joint to move without friction.

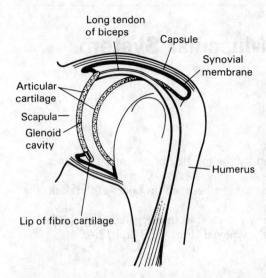

Fig. 12.3 The shoulder joint (diagrammatic section). The upper end or head of the humerus is seen fitting into the glenoid cavity or socket of the scapula. The ligaments are thickened portions of the capsule.

This cartilage is thickest in the centre of the joint, and because it is slightly elastic tends to reduce jarring. The two ends of the bone are connected by the joint capsule, which is formed of white fibrous tissue. This capsule is thickened and reinforced by ligaments which vary in strength and position, depending on the position of the joint. These add stability, and by their position restrain the joint from making abnormal movements. The ligaments will be described with regard to individual joints.

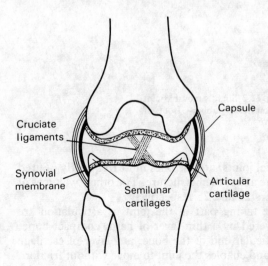

Fig. 12.4 The knee joint (diagrammatic section). The lower end of the femur is seen articulating with the upper end of the tibia. Note: the ligaments are thickened parts of the capsule.

The inner aspect of the capsule is lined with the synovial membrane, which is a thick membrane attached to the articular edges of the bone and to the capsule, and receiving a rich blood supply. This membrane secretes the synovial fluid which lubricates the inside of the joint.

Each joint receives a rich nerve supply to the synovia, capsule, ligaments and bones. These sensory nerves enable the brain to locate the exact position of the joint and to assess stretch in the ligaments or capsule, and also carry pain fibres. The nerves which supply the muscles of the joint always send a sensory branch to the inside of the joint. This enables movements to be carefully coordinated. The rich sensory supply, however, makes the joint extremely sensitive; pain will be felt even with slight damage, and the reflex spasm of the muscles will restrict movement.

The long bones articulate by their ends, the flat by their edges and the short by various parts of their surfaces.

Movements of joints

These are gliding, angular, rotatory or circumductory. The gliding consists of a simple sliding of the apposed surfaces of the bones, one upon another, without angular or rotatory motion. It is common to all movable joints, and is the only kind of movement possible between the individual small bones of the wrist and foot. Angular movement occurs at the hinge joints, and the range of movement is restricted by the ligaments or bony configuration of the joint. Angular movements are flexion to bend the joint and extension to straighten the joint. Rotatory movements occur in ball and socket joints, the turning of a bone upon a vertical axis. Ball and socket joints also allow flexion and extension to occur and, in addition, adduction where the limb is moved to the body and abduction where the limb is moved away from the body. A combination of all these is seen in circumductory movements.

The muscular system

Muscles are the meat of the body. They act on bones to move them or, as in the trunk, to protect and support the organs within the body. Muscle is made up of individual fibres, the size and number of which vary depending upon their position in the body and the size of the muscle as a whole. Exercise can increase the size of the individual fibre and thus the size of the muscle, but the number of fibres remains constant.

Muscles are attached to bone, either by connective tissue, tendon, or a combination of these. These attachments are extremely strong and either the muscle or the tendon will tear rather than be pulled from the bone directly.

Individual muscle fibres have a thin layer of fibrous tissue around them. Bundles of muscle fibres and muscles also have coverings of fibrous tissue which thicken in certain positions and are called fascia. The amount of fibrous tissue within a muscle varies. When a muscle contracts and shortens, one end usually remains stationary: this is called the origin of the muscle. The other end, drawn up by the contraction of the muscle, is called the insertion of the muscle (see Fig. 12.5). The nerve to a muscle carries impulses which cause it to contract. This is the motor part of the nerve supply; individual nerve fibres may supply from 5 to 150 muscle fibres, and there is a considerable overlap. This allows very precise movements to take place.

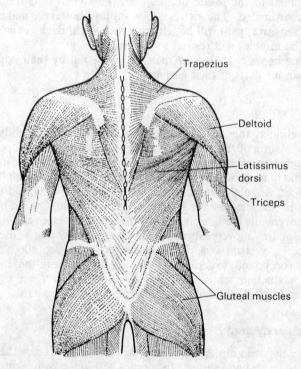

Fig. 12.5 The superficial muscles of the back and limbs. Note the origins of the muscles, e.g. the deltoid from the scapula, and how it tapers towards its insertion on the humerus.

The muscle fibre converts circulating glucose and oxygen into energy, and produces carbon dioxide and lactic acid (see Chapter 14). The efficiency of the muscle in dealing with the waste products is improved by regular exercise. A good blood supply is important, and this is also increased during muscular activities. However, sometimes during increased activity an 'oxygen debt' is built up (anaerobic metabolism). The waste products accumulate and the muscle feels pain and cramp.

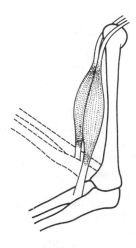

Fig. 12.6 Diagrammatic representation of action of biceps. Dotted lines show changes on muscle contraction.

Movements

All movements are carefully coordinated: when one muscle contracts the opposing muscle or muscle group is gradually relaxing (Fig. 12.6). This produces a smooth movement without jerking. Regular practice, e.g. sports, gymnastics or ballet, will improve this coordination and at the same time improve the state of the muscle and produce more power and agility.

Types of muscle action

Prime movers play the major part in moving the joint.

Muscles of fixation produce a stable base for the movement of limbs or other muscles.

Group synergists give indirect assistance and a steadying effect on the prime movers.

Specialized forms of muscles are seen in the heart and in the walls of the organs of the body, the stomach, bowel and bladder. These are not under the voluntary control of the body but respond to the autonomic nervous system (see Chapter 10).

13

The Digestive System

Digestion is the conversion of foodstuffs into simple substances which can be easily absorbed into the blood-stream. The digestive system consists of:

1. The alimentary canal, the passage along which food passes while digestion is taking place. The alimentary canal is nearly 9 metres long and leads through the body from the mouth to the anus.

2. The digestive glands. These secrete liquids which enter the alimentary canal. The liquids contain substances called enzymes which act upon the various foodstuffs, converting them into simple products.

When food is taken into the mouth it is masticated and thoroughly mixed with saliva. Saliva is secreted by a number of glands situated near the mouth; it contains a valuable enzyme for the breakdown of starches, moistens the food, and acts as a lubricant.

After mastication the food is rolled up into a small ball, called a bolus, ready for swallowing. Swallowing is not completely under the control of the will, and once it has begun it cannot be stopped. This is a protective mechanism which prevents food from finding its way into the air passages.

From the back of the tongue the bolus is passed through the pharynx and enters the oesophagus, the opening of which relaxes to receive it. The oesophagus is a long, thin tube which connects the pharynx to the stomach. It passes down the back of the neck and thoracic cavity, lying behind the heart and great blood vessels; it then pierces the diaphragm and opens into the stomach, which is the first digestive organ within the abdomen (see Fig. 13.1).

Stomach. This is a bag-like organ, made of muscle and lined by mucous membrane. It is situated in the upper part of the abdomen, lying chiefly on the left side. The main function of the stomach is to store food. Only small quantities at a time can be passed into the duodenum.

When a meal enters the stomach, digestion begins actively, and, owing to the continuous waves of contraction and relaxation of the stomach muscles, the food is mixed with other digestive juices secreted by the mucous membrane itself. This churning continues as long as there is any food left in the stomach; this may last as long as three hours after a full meal, but some of the food begins to leave the stomach within half an hour.

The stomach leads into the duodenum, which is the first part of the small intestine, and the food is mixed with digestive juices secreted by the liver, the pancreas and the intestines themselves.

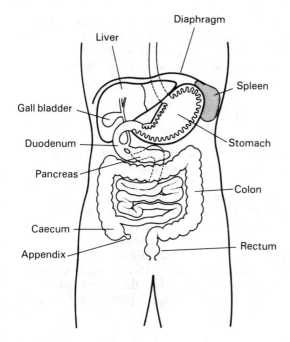

Diaphragm

Liver

Gall bladder

Duodenum

Pancreas

Caecum

Appendix

Spleen

Stomach

Colon

Rectum

Fig. 13.1 The digestive system.

From the duodenum the alimentary canal continues as the small intestine. This is a muscular tube lined by mucous membrane, about 7 m in length. Except for the first 25 cm, the small intestine is folded upon itself to form coils which fit neatly into the abdominal cavity.

The food is forced along the intestine by waves of muscular contraction called peristalsis; during this journey digestion is completed and most of the nutrients are absorbed into the blood-stream.

About four and a half hours after the commencement of the meal, such food products as have not already been absorbed are nearing the end of the small intestine and are beginning to enter the large intestine or colon.

Colon. This is about 1.5 m long and of a much larger diameter than the small intestine. It begins, as the caecum, in the lower part of the right side of the abdomen; to the caecum is attached the appendix.

From the caecum the colon travels upwards to the liver (ascending colon), where it takes a bend and crosses over to the left side (transverse colon); it then make a second bend near the spleen and descends along the left side into the lower part of the abdomen (descending colon). From here it is continued as an S-shaped loop (sigmoid colon) which joins the rectum.

Few food products are absorbed from the colon but large quantities of water are taken up into the blood; for this reason the contents of the colon tend to become more and more solid as they proceed along its course. The unabsorbed remnants of the meal, together with intestinal juices, are evacuated from the rectum as faeces.

Peritoneum. The abdomen is lined by the peritoneum, which is a serous glistening membrane with a good blood supply. This provides, in addition, an outer coat or covering for the intestines.

The small intestine is attached to the posterior wall of the abdomen by a relatively small double fold of peritoneum known as the mesentery. This spreads out fanwise from its attachment at the back of the abdomen and acts as a sling, preventing the small intestine from dropping downwards into the pelvis. In a wound of the abdomen, coils of small intestine may find their way to the exterior and will be recognized by their greyish-white glistening appearance, which is caused by their outer coat of peritoneum.

The colon is also invested with peritoneum, but only certain parts possess a mesentery. For this reason the colon is less mobile than the small intestine.

The peritoneum serves to prevent friction when the abdominal organs move on one another; it also carries blood vessels, lymphatics and nerves to the various organs.

Other organs within the abdomen

Besides the alimentary canal and a number of large blood vessels, the abdomen contains several important organs; a few of these must be briefly described.

The liver. This is the largest gland in the body and weighs about 1.5 kg. It is of a dark reddish-brown colour and contains a large quantity of blood. It is situated in the upper part of the abdomen beneath the diaphragm. The liver is divided into two main lobes, of which the right is much larger than the left.

The liver has many functions, including storing glucose and secreting bile, a thick greenish-yellow fluid which plays an important part in digestion. Blood from the gut drains via the portal vein to the liver, where the food products are removed. The blood then enters the general circulation via the hepatic veins.

Bile is conveyed from the right and left lobes of the liver by two channels, which join each other and form a tube which ultimately opens into the duodenum. This duct gives off a branch which leads to the gallbladder, a small pear-shaped organ situated on the under surface of the right lobe of the liver. The gallbladder stores bile when it is not required in the alimentary canal.

The pancreas. This is an important gland which lies across the back of the abdomen behind the stomach. (See Fig. 13.1.)

The pancreas secretes a digestive fluid which is conveyed along a duct to the duodenum. It also produces a hormone called insulin; this enters the blood stream directly and enables the tissues to utilize the glucose which is brought to them by the blood. Deficiency of insulin causes the disease called diabetes mellitus, or simply diabetes.

The spleen. This is a small organ of a deep purplish-red colour. It is situated on the left side of the upper abdomen, under the lower ribs and behind the stomach.

The spleen is a source of white blood corpuscles (which are concerned with immunity) and also destroys red corpuscles which have become worn out.

The urinary system

This is also situated within the abdomen and pelvis. It consists of the kidneys, the ureters, the bladder and the urethra (Fig. 13.2).

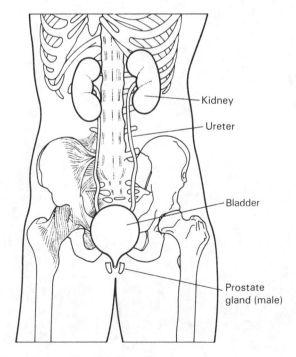

Fig. 13.2 The urinary system.

The kidneys are situated high up on the back of the abdominal cavity, one on either side of the spinal column; the right kidney lies a little lower than the left.

The kidneys remove waste products from the blood. These waste products are secreted as urine, which leaves the kidneys and drains into the ureters.

The ureters are two fine tubes, running from each kidney to the bladder. They are from 25 to 30 cm long and about 0.25 cm thick. They run down the back of the abdomen, enter the pelvis, and terminate by entering the bladder.

The bladder is a muscular bag which acts as a reservoir for the urine. It lies to the front of the pelvic cavity.

The urethra is the passage leading from the bladder to the outer surface of the body.

14

Foodstuffs, Metabolism and Body Temperature

NUTRIENTS AND METABOLISM

The body's requirements for nutrients are:
1. Water.
2. Carbohydrates.
3. Fats.
4. Protein.
5. Vitamins.
6. Minerals.
It is able to store some of these substances for long periods, others for a very short time only.

Water

Although some water is produced by metabolism (burning of food as fuel), losses are such that one needs to drink a variable amount each day: this should be about three pints (1500 ml) on an average day, but more would be required on a hot day or after heavy exercise.

Carbohydrates

Those found in food are largely sugars and starch. Substances (enzymes) in saliva and pancreatic secretion break down the complex sugars into simpler ones. The eventual end product is glucose. Following a meal, a large amount of glucose is absorbed. It cannot all be used at once, so some is stored as a 'complex sugar' (similar to starch) called glycogen, or converted to fat. This store of glycogen is called upon during short periods of starvation, for example overnight. When reserves of glycogen are used up the body must rely on its reserves of fat and protein for energy production (Fig. 14.1).

If enough oxygen is available, for example at rest or during moderate exercise, pathway 1 is used. This is called **aerobic metabolism**. However, if not enough oxygen is available, less energy is produced, and lactic acid is formed by **anaerobic metabolism** illustrated in pathway 2. The build up of lactic acid fatigues the muscles, thus limiting exercise.

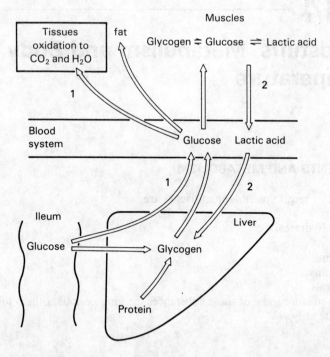

Fig. 14.1 Production of energy.

Fats

Dietary fats are also broken down by the digestive processes and absorbed as simpler molecules (Fig. 14.2).

Protein

The 'building blocks' of proteins are amino acids. It is in this form that protein material is absorbed after digestion. Amino acids are used to build new body proteins, but can also be used (if surplus to requirements or in starvation) to produce energy (Fig. 14.3).

Vitamins

These are essential in the chemical processes which take place in the cell. Vitamin K, for example, is important in the manufacture of the 'clotting factors' which coagulate the blood.

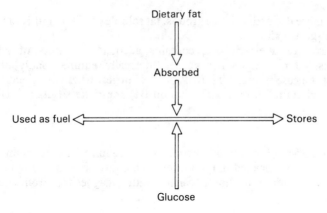

Fig. 14.2 Fat metabolism.

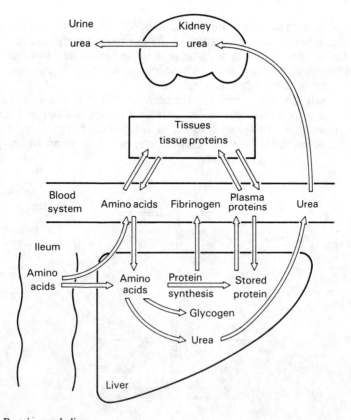

Fig. 14.3 Protein metabolism.

Vitamins are divided into two groups: fat soluble (A, D, E and K) and water soluble (B-group and C).

The average Western diet contains adequate amounts of all these substances. Vitamin supplements are not normally required. Sadly, however, this is not the case in many Third World countries, where deficiencies result in scurvy (vitamin C), beri-beri (vitamin B1) and rickets (vitamin D).

Minerals

A large number of different chemicals are required to maintain health, although some are needed only in minute amounts. The most important are potassium, sodium, phosphorus, calcium, zinc, magnesium, iron, cobalt and copper.

REGULATION OF BODY TEMPERATURE

Humans, being mammals, are 'warm blooded'. That is to say that, despite wide variations in the temperature of the environment, their core temperature is maintained by balancing heat production against heat loss (Fig. 14.4). ('Cold blooded' animals, such as reptiles, cannot do this and assume the temperature of their surroundings.)

The body must maintain the temperature of the vital organs (the core temperature) to within narrow limits in order to ensure optimal function. Other areas of the body, such as the skin (the periphery), may be several degrees cooler than the core temperature, which is approximately 37°C

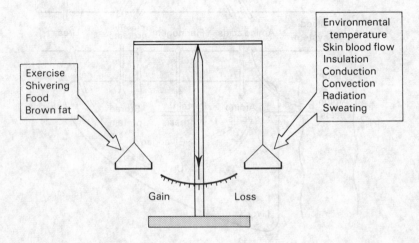

Fig. 14.4 Heat gain versus heat loss.

(98.6°F). This temperature varies by small amounts (plus or minus one degree) in healthy individuals.

Heat production

The main source of heat is skeletal muscle, which during exercise releases a considerable proportion of the energy obtained by 'burning' glucose in the form of heat. Much less heat is produced when at rest. In the adult, the contribution from metabolism varies little. As the ambient temperature falls, warm blooded animals begin to shiver. This increases heat production by contracting the skeletal muscle. A special form of fat, called 'brown fat', can be quickly mobilized to produce extra heat when required. This is rather like switching on a heater. Brown fat occurs in humans and other mammals.

Heat loss

Heat may be lost by the body through
- (a) conduction,
- (b) convection, and
- (c) radiation (the greatest proportion).

Heat loss may be **decreased** by **insulation** (fur, hair, clothes). **Sweating**, however, **increases** heat loss, by taking the heat required to evaporate the sweat from the body itself, which correspondingly cools. This mechanism is the main defence against the body temperature becoming too high (hyperthermia). Babies are unable to control their body temperature very well in adverse environments: for example a small baby left naked in a cold room will rapidly lose heat (become hypothermic).

Mechanisms activated by cold

1. Shivering.
2. Hunger.   } Increased heat production.
3. Increased activity.
4. Reduction in skin blood flow.   } Decreased heat loss.
5. Erection of hair.

Mechanisms activated by heat

1. Increased skin blood flow
   (increased radiation).
2. Sweating.   } Increased heat loss.
3. Increased respiration (panting)
   leading to increased evaporation.
4. Loss of appetite.   } Reduced heat production.
5. Decreased activity.

Fever

This special state occurs when the body temperature is maintained at a higher level than normal ('the thermostat is reset'). It is a defence mechanism in response to infection and toxins.

Causes of a raised body temperature (hyperthermia):

1. Fever (due to infections, etc.); heat stroke.
2. Excess insulation (in babies and infants, often due to too much clothing).
3. Head injuries.
4. Certain tumours.
5. Thyroid disease.
6. Atropine (belladonna) poisoning.

Causes of abnormally low body temperature (hypothermia):

1. Accidental hypothermia (particularly in the elderly).
2. Immersion in cold water (see below).
3. Thyroid disease.
4. Some poisonings, e.g. barbiturates.

Immersion

Upon exposure to cold (for example, immersion in cold water) the blood vessels in the skin dilate and heat is lost from the core to the periphery very quickly. It is important to realize that many victims of 'drowning' are in fact suffering cold injury.

Part 3
Clinical Practice

— 15

Asphyxia and Respiratory Disorders

Asphyxia means that not enough oxygen is reaching the body tissues. Irreversible brain damage will occur within three to five minutes at normal body temperature if the brain is completely deprived of oxygen. This interval is, however, prolonged if the core temperature is low – for example, following immersion in cold water.

The causes may be grouped as follows:
1. Inadequate ventilation of the lungs.
2. Inadequate oxygen in the inspired air.
3. Interference with the transport and utilization of oxygen.

CAUSES OF ASPHYXIA

Inadequate ventilation

This may be the result of any of the following:
1. Obstructed airway (Fig. 15.1) caused by
   (a) the tongue falling back in the unconscious casualty,
   (b) vomit, dentures, food or other inhaled foreign body,
   (c) bee or wasp stings affecting the throat or airway,
   (d) swelling from burns and scalds or inhalation of toxic chemicals,
   (e) strangulation or hanging,
   (f) neck injuries.
2. Suffocation, due to
   (a) plastic bags being placed over the heads of children, or babies being placed face down on a pillow, or
   (b) being trapped in an airtight cupboard, box or refrigerator.
3. Compression of the chest, caused by
   (a) a collapsing building or trench, or
   (b) crush injury in a traffic accident or crowd.
4. Blast injuries.
5. Fluid in the lungs, due to
   (a) heart failure, or
   (b) inhalation of toxic chemicals or smoke.
6. Electrocution.
7. Epileptic fits.

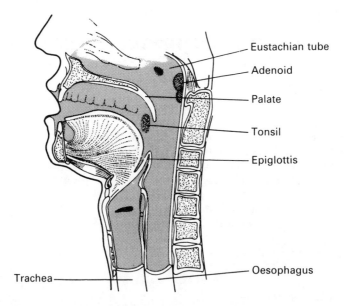

Fig. 15.1 Section through the nasal passages, mouth, pharynx, etc.

8. Damage to the nervous system, caused by
    (a) spinal injury or
    (b) stroke.
9. Poisoning.
10. Bronchospasm (asthma).

Inadequate oxygen in the inspired air

This condition may occur in the following circumstances:
1. Inhalation of smoke or fumes, or gas leaks.
2. High altitudes, occurring
    (a) when climbing to high altitudes, or
    (b) during decompression in aircraft.
3. Diving accidents
4. Drowning.

Interference with the transport and utilization of oxygen

1. Transport, e.g. carbon monoxide poisoning.
2. Utilization, e.g. cyanide poisoning.

Symptoms and signs of respiratory distress

1. Increased respiratory effort.
2. Indrawing of muscle between the ribs (in respiratory obstruction).
3. Cyanosis.
4. Deteriorating conscious level.
5. Eventual respiratory and cardiac arrest.

Treatment

General principles of the treatment of respiratory disorders

If possible, remove the cause of the problem (or the casualty from the cause) **but remember your own safety.**

SPECIFIC CONDITIONS

Inhaled foreign body (choking)

The foreign body is commonly food in adults, but may well be small objects such as peanuts, beads or pen tops in children. A small foreign body may pass down into the lung without causing obstruction until it reaches a small bronchus. It may not cause any trouble there for some time, coming to light only later with partial collapse of the lung and infection. There may be a chronic cough, due to irritation of the bronchial wall, and production of excess secretions.

Larger foreign bodies may impact at the vocal cords or in one of the main bronchi. If the object is lodged in the larynx or trachea, complete respiratory obstruction may ensue.

Symptoms and signs

1. Respiratory distress.
2. Coughing and choking.
3. Congestion of the face.
4. Cyanosis.
5. Cessation of breathing.
6. Unconsciousness.
7. Eventual cardiac arrest.

Treatment

Back blows. Strike the casualty between the shoulder blades with the heel of the hand. Encourage coughing and keep the patient bent forwards. Check after each blow to see if there has been any improvement. If this treatment is unsuccessful after several blows, the Heimlich manoeuvre or abdominal thrust should be attempted (see below).

For children or unconscious victims. Place the casualty over the rescuer's knees if possible to perform the blows. Smaller children require less force, but children over 14 years old should be treated as adults.

For infants. The rescuer should sit and hold the infant's body, **supported**, almost upside down with one arm and hand, making sure that the head is supported. The blows are applied by slapping with the **fingers** of the other hand.

Note. If the casualty has stopped breathing or is cyanosed (blue lips), attempt artificial respiration at once between the blows. In some cases, the obstruction may be moved forward (into a main bronchus) by the rescuer's respiratory effort. In this case, only one lung will be obstructed and the casualty should recover, as adequate ventilation should be possible with the other lung.

Heimlich manoeuvre. The principle behind this method of treatment is that compression of the upper abdomen will force the diaphragm upwards, expelling any residual air in the lungs. This may dislodge the foreign body by an 'artificial cough'.

For adults and larger children. The rescuer stands behind the patient and clasps his hands together at the point of the 'solar plexus' (X in Fig. 15.2). Both hands are then pulled firmly upward. This may be repeated several times.

Note. Incorrect placement of the hands may cause organ damage, for example, to liver, spleen or stomach.

Unconscious victims. The casualty should be placed supine on a firm surface. The rescuer sits astride the victim and positions his hands as for cardiac massage (the heel of one hand upon the other) **but over the solar plexus.** The abdomen is then compressed by the rescuer rocking forward with his arms held straight.

Smaller children. Only one hand (with the fist clenched) is required in children under about six years of age. The manoeuvre is performed in the same way as for adults, with the rescuer kneeling or with the child on his lap (Fig. 15.3).

Infants. The child should be placed supine on a firm surface. The abdomen is relatively large in babies and the position for compression differs slightly

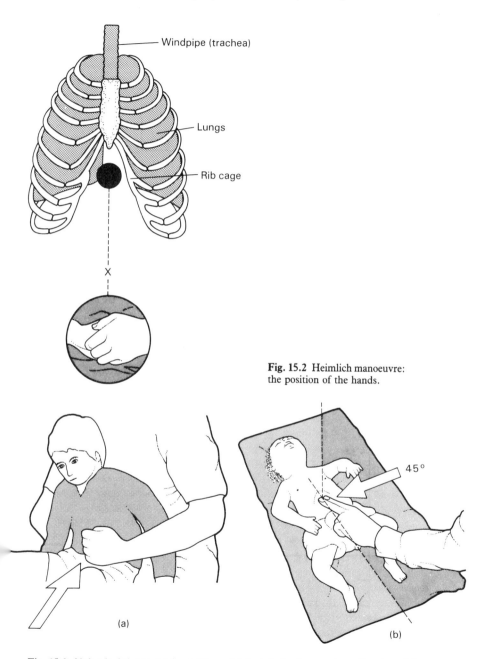

Fig. 15.2 Heimlich manoeuvre: the position of the hands.

Windpipe (trachea)

Lungs

Rib cage

X

45°

(a)

(b)

Fig. 15.3 Abdominal thrust: (a) for children; (b) for infants. Arrows show direction of thrust.

from that in adults. **Two fingers only** should be used, placed two-thirds of the way between the umbilicus (navel) and the point where the rib margins meet. Firm thrusts at forty-five degrees should then be made (Fig. 15.3). If the infant coughs and the obstruction appears to be moving, the manoeuvre should be followed up with back blows as above.

Crush injury to the chest

This may be the result of being crushed, for example, by a vehicle, by falling masonry, or in a crowd. The main problem is disruption of the bony rib cage, making respiration difficult and painful. In addition, the damaged ribs may tear the lung or pleura: leakage of air under the skin produces swelling which crackles on pressure, i.e. surgical emphysema. If the ribs are broken in more than one place along their length, a 'flail segment' results which displays 'paradoxical respiration', moving in the opposite way to the rest of the chest wall (e.g., it is sucked in on inspiration) (Fig. 15.4). This results in collapse of the lung on the affected side.

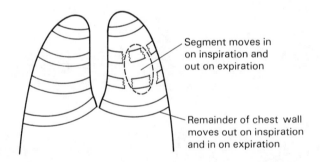

Segment moves in
on inspiration and
out on expiration

Remainder of chest wall
moves out on inspiration
and in on expiration

Fig. 15.4 Diagrammatic representation of a 'flail segment'.

A 'sucking wound' may be caused by a stab or missile injury or even (rarely) by a fractured rib. In such a wound, air enters the chest through the wound on inspiration and bubbles of frothy blood appear on expiration.

Air may enter through such a wound, but be unable to leave due to a 'flap–valve' effect resulting in air accumulating under tension within the chest cavity. The pressure may displace the heart into the 'good' side of the chest and may ultimately compress the 'good' lung. This is an extremely dangerous condition which must be treated early to avoid a fatality.

Symptoms and signs

1. Respiratory distress.
2. Paradoxical respiration.
3. The presence of a 'sucking wound' bubbling blood.
4. Bloodstained, frothy sputum being coughed up.

Treatment

1. Cover any wound with something airtight, for example a plastic bag, taped in place if possible. A pad and bandage (shell dressing – see Chapter 34) is effective in larger wounds.
2. Support the rib cage where it shows paradoxical respiration, with a hand across the flail segment.
3. Incline the casualty to the **injured** side to promote maximum movement in the normal side.
4. Strap the casualty's arm across the injured chest to stabilize it (Fig. 15.5).
5. Call an ambulance as soon as possible.

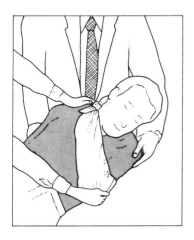

Fig. 15.5 Treatment of crush injury to the chest. Casualty inclined to the injured side.

Electrocution

This may be divided into low-voltage and high-voltage injury. The latter group includes lightning strikes.

Low voltage electrocution. By this we mean voltages up to and including that of the mains supply (220–240V AC in the UK). A rescuer will be safe providing that he does not touch the casualty with bare hands or with anything wet. Low voltage injuries may cause burns, but the main danger is from cardiac arrest. Respiration may be impossible because the passage of the electric current holds the muscles contracted. For this reason, even a conscious casualty may be unable to break free from the live conductor.

High voltage electrocution. The high voltages found in overhead transmission lines are of the order of 33 000 to 400 000 volts. Contact causes immediate cardiac arrest and severe disruption of tissue due to the heating effect of the electric current as it passes through the body. Violent muscular contraction may throw the casualty clear of the point of contact.

It is not safe to approach such a situation since the high voltage may arc to earth over a distance of many metres. One can do nothing for such a casualty until the electricity has been turned off.

By then it is unlikely that resuscitation will be possible.

Lightning injury. A lightning bolt may be charged to over a million volts, but the current flow is of very short duration. If a person is hit he may suffer cardiac arrest, but this is not always the case. Severe burns may occur at the point of entry and exit of the current. In addition, the victim's clothes may be set on fire.

Signs of electrocution

1. Pallor or cyanosis.
2. Absent respiration.
3. Evidence of contact with electricity.
4. Unconsciousness.

Treatment

Low voltage injury

1. Break the contact by switching off the current, preferably at the main switch. If this is impracticable, remove the plug or switch off at the appliance. If this cannot be done, stand on a **dry** insulator such as a doormat, and using a dry piece of wood or other insulator, separate the casualty from the live conductor. **Never use anything containing metal for this purpose.**
2. Commence resuscitation.
3. Treat for shock (lay the patient down and raise the legs at the hip; place pillows or cushions under the knees).
4. Summon an ambulance.
5. Treat burns.

High voltage injury

No useful first aid treatment can be given until the electricity has been switched off. Thereafter, it will consist of resuscitation and treatment for burns. In contrast to power line injuries, lightning strikes are of such short duration that resuscitation is often successful. The burns are deep.

Inhalation of smoke or fumes

Because fire consumes the oxygen in its vicinity, the casualty is likely to be suffering from direct oxygen lack as well as from the toxic effects of the smoke. Many modern articles of furniture produce cyanide gas as they burn. The smoke may be a strong irritant to the airway, resulting in spasm of the vocal cords and damage to the lining of the respiratory tract. Gas leaks may fill the room with gas, displacing the oxygen.

Symptoms and signs

1. Coughing; watering of the eyes.
2. Difficulty with respiration; cyanosis.
3. Unconsciousness.
4. Respiratory and cardiac arrest.
5. Burns.
6. Shock.

Treatment

1. **If it is safe to do so**, remove the casualty from the situation. Do not fight the fire.
2. If clothing is on fire, wrap the victim in a blanket to extinguish the flames.
3. Artificial respiration (together with cardiac massage if there is no pulse).
4. Call the emergency services.

Decompression

At high altitude

The amount of oxygen available to the body decreases as the barometric pressure falls with high altitude. An aircraft flying at 30 000 feet normally has sufficient cabin pressure to provide an environment equivalent to only a few hundred feet of altitude. If there is sudden decompression, there will be insufficient oxygen available to even maintain consciousness, which will be lost within minutes. Modern aircraft are equipped with an oxygen supply, and masks which are deployed automatically in the event of depressurization.

Note: patients with heart and lung disease may be unable to tolerate even the short time it takes to deploy the oxygen masks in such an event, and may suffer chest pain or even cardiac arrest.

Diving accidents

Decompression problems may affect divers who return to the surface too quickly, or who are evacuated by air transport after any other sort of accident following a dive. If the diver has been breathing air under pressure (whilst diving), nitrogen becomes dissolved in his body fluids in increased amounts. If he decompresses too quickly, **or subsequently ascends to altitude,** the nitrogen may come out of solution to form bubbles in the blood stream, lungs, bone and brain. This leads to pain, respiratory distress, clouding of consciousness and loss of balance (variously described as 'the bends', 'the chokes', 'the narks' etc.).

Urgent *expert* treatment is required

Treatment

First aid treatment consists of:
1. Descent to near sea level if flying.
2. Reassurance and prevention of exertion.
3. Allow divers access to oxygen if they are familiar with the apparatus.
4. Summon expert help via the police or ambulance service.
The only effective treatment lies in transfer to a pressure chamber once the above measures have been carried out.

Drowning

Well-documented attempts at resuscitation of the drowned casualty are to be found in the writings of antiquity but modern interest in the subject began in the 1740s. A case of successful resuscitation by the mouth-to-mouth method was reported in 1744! Drowning is an increasingly common occurrence with the growing popularity of water sports. Hypothermia (see Chapter 14) very frequently accompanies drowning, and many of those who have drowned have, in fact, become unconscious from hypothermia and subsequently inhaled water.

Survival following immersion in water depends upon many factors, the most important of which are water temperature, physical fitness, ability to swim, insulation (clothes or wet suit) and distance from land.

Drowning begins when the victim is no longer able to keep his mouth and nose above the water. Initially, most of the water entering the mouth is swallowed. This may provoke vomiting and stomach contents may be inhaled, causing asphyxia.

Dry drowning. Asphyxia in these cases is due to intense spasm (sustained contraction) of the vocal cords. If rescued in time, however, the spasm may be 'broken' by giving mouth-to-mouth resuscitation. In any event, the spasm will become less severe with the passage of time as the muscles are deprived of oxygen. Death may occur instantaneously, however, due to reflex cardiac arrest caused by contact of the larynx with the inhaled water. Cases of 'dry' drowning are thought to form between 10 and 40 per cent of all cases.

Wet drowning. In this form of drowning, water enters the lungs. No attempt should be made to remove it. Fresh water drowning results in more rapid death from cardiac arrest than salt water drowning, because fresh water (containing few dissolved salts) passes more rapidly into the cells causing them to swell and burst. The process releases large quantities of potassium, which is responsible for the cardiac arrest.

Symptoms and signs

1. Respiratory distress or absent respiration.
2. Cyanosis.
3. Unconsciousness.
4. Production of frothy sputum.

Treatment

1. Artificial ventilation, in the water if necessary.
2. Recovery position, when normal respiration has been restored.
3. Prevention of hypothermia.
4. Call an ambulance.

Carbon monoxide poisoning

Carbon monoxide is colourless and has no smell. **It may kill without warning.** It is produced in car exhausts and by incomplete combustion in, for example, gas and coal fires. **Natural gas appliances can still kill through carbon monoxide poisoning** (due to incomplete combustion).

Carbon monoxide is bound more readily than is oxygen to the haemoglobin in the blood. It prevents oxygen from combining with haemoglobin, thus effectively preventing it from being transported to the tissues.

Symptoms and signs

1. Signs of asphyxia (**remember that in such cases the casualty will remain pink**, as the combination of carbon monoxide with haemoglobin produces a cherry pink colour).
2. Confusion and clouding of consciousness.

Note: the first aider must **never** enter a gas-filled room alone. **You cannot smell or see carbon monoxide and loss of consciousness may be sudden.**

If it is not possible to open the windows and doors or remove the casualty without taking a breath, it is better for the first aider not to attempt a rescue but to wait for the fire brigade. If the first aider does decide to enter the room, he should tie a lifeline around his waist and maintain tension on it with an assistant outside. Loss of tension will indicate that he is in difficulties.

Many would-be rescuers have died through being overcome by fumes in an attempt to rescue others. It is important not to take a breath whilst inside the room.

This principle also applies to empty tanks which have contained petrol, fuel oil or dry-cleaning fluid.

Treatment

1. Remove from the source of carbon monoxide.
2. Artificial ventilation.

Cyanide poisoning

Cyanide gas is produced during the combustion of modern plastic materials. It is also found as a solid chemical, e.g. as potassium cyanide, in industry. Cyanide prevents the utilization of energy produced within the cell from the metabolism of glucose. Swallowing the solid chemical is usually fatal unless in minute amounts, as is inhaling any quantity of cyanide gas. Apart from standard resuscitation, there is no effective first aid treatment. Industrial users of cyanide should be familiar with the use of antidotes which are beyond the scope of the first aider.

Other chest injuries

Blast injury

Injuries from a bomb or gas explosion, for example, are usually multiple and often involve the chest. Ribs may be fractured with the production of a flail segment. Treatment is as for the crush injuries to the chest discussed above. In addition, blast injury damages the airway and alveoli, resulting in impaired transfer of oxygen into the blood stream and an outpouring of bloodstained fluid into the alveoli. Urgent expert help is required.

Missile and stab wounds

Missiles such as shrapnel, bullets and flying debris from collapsing buildings, etc., may cause a pneumothorax if they penetrate the chest wall. The resulting 'sucking wound' should be treated in the same manner as one caused by the penetration of a fractured rib through the pleural membrane described above. High velocity missile injuries may cause very severe disruption of tissue inside the chest cavity.

Diaphragmatic injuries

Blunt trauma to the abdomen may result in rupture of the diaphragm. The bowel and other abdominal contents may then enter the chest, compressing the lungs and causing severe respiratory distress. Treatment should follow that indicated above, under 'general principles' of the treatment of respiratory disorders.

Injuries to the heart and major blood vessels

Any major chest trauma, especially direct blunt injury to the front of the chest or a penetrating injury, may result in severe blood loss due to damage to the heart or vessels in the chest. Accumulation of blood in the pericardial sac prevents the heart from filling properly and may severely reduce the cardiac output and blood pressure. Death may occur within seconds from haemorrhage if the heart or major vessels are torn. Cardiac arrest may occur from a severe direct blow to the chest. Treatment relies on the general principles of treatment for shock and cardiopulmonary resuscitation.

RESPIRATORY DISORDERS

Respiratory disorders may be divided into those which have been present for a long time and those which have occurred suddenly. Those which have been present for a long time will usually have resulted in the patient seeking medical advice, resulting in many cases in the prescription of some medication by the doctor. Of this group, exacerbations of asthma are of particular note to first aiders.

Asthma

The patient is often a child, but the disease affects both adults and children. Some patients have a nervous predisposition and are highly 'strung', but most have an allergic response to contact with certain substances such as house dust.

The walls of the air passages (bronchi) contain muscle. During an attack of asthma the muscle is in spasm (sustained contraction), which narrows the airways so much that it is difficult for air to pass into or out of the lung.

It is important to remember that most asthmatics are used to coping with an attack. They are often taking medicines on a regular basis in an attempt to prevent attacks occurring. However, particularly severe attacks may cause extreme respiratory distress and exhaustion, and are very frightening.

Symptoms and signs

1. A frightened, sweating patient very short of breath. There is particular difficulty in breathing out.
2. Extra muscular effort is visible as the patient attempts to breathe. He or she tends to sit upright.
3. There may be cyanosis. This is a serious sign.

Treatment

1. Reassurance.
2. Encourage the patient to sit with his elbows resting on a table. This ensures maximum mechanical advantage for the muscles which aid respiration.
3. If the patient has his medicine with him, encourage him to take it **but not repeatedly.** Medication usually takes the form of an inhaler but may be syrup or tablets.
4. Call for medical help if symptoms do not quickly subside, or if there is cyanosis.

Disorders of sudden onset

The most life-threatening of these are dealt with above, under asphyxia. Others include the following.

Pneumonia

This is a bacterial or viral infection of the lungs. It usually only affects one side at a time. The inflammation may spread to the pleura (pleurisy) and thick secretions containing pus may be coughed up.

Symptoms and signs

1. Fever and malaise. The patient may shiver uncontrollably (rigor).
2. Pain in the chest. If the pleura is involved the pain will be worse on inspiration.
3. Cough with production of rusty coloured or yellow sputum.

Treatment

1. Keep the patient warm and at rest, preferably in bed.
2. Seek medical attention.

Coughing of blood

This used to be commonly seen when tuberculosis (TB) was prevalent, but is rare nowadays. It should always be taken seriously, especially following an accident when damage to the lung may have occurred.

Treatment

1. Reassurance.
2. Call for urgent medical assistance.

Spontaneous collapse of a lung (pneumothorax)

This tends to occur in fit young adults. The cause is usually an inherited weakness in the pleura overlying the lung which, when it ruptures, allows air to enter the chest cavity with resultant collapse of the lung. It may also occur in certain chronic lung diseases.

Symptoms and signs

1. Sudden onset of pain in the chest.
2. Shortness of breath.
Respiration is usually not severely affected, as the remaining lung, if healthy, can cope while the patient is at rest.

Treatment

1. Reassurance.
2. Seek medical attention.

The common cold and influenza

Most of us have experienced these conditions. Influenza, however, may make the patient feel very unwell and even unable to stand. Pneumonia may follow such an illness, and before the coming of antibiotics was responsible for many deaths (as in the epidemic of 1918).

Treatment

1. Bed rest.
2. Encourage fluids.
3. Aspirin or paracetamol to relieve aches and fever.
4. If persistent cough productive of sputum develops, seek medical advice.

Hiccough

This is due to premature contraction of the diaphragm. Only rarely is the condition persistent.

Treatment

The attack can usually be terminated by raising the amount of carbon dioxide in the blood. This is best achieved by asking the patient to breathe from a **paper** (not plastic) bag for a few minutes.

Note: under no circumstances should a plastic bag be employed. During this manoeuvre the patient should not be left alone.

Winding

A blow to the upper abdomen ('solar plexus') forces the casualty to exhale and results in subsequent shortness of breath for a few moments. There may be associated nausea and vomiting.

Treatment

1. Reassurance.
2. Loosen all clothing around the neck and chest.
3. Massaging the abdomen may help.
4. If the casualty vomits, ensure that none is inhaled.

— 16

Cardiac and Circulatory Problems

The major pulses

A pulse follows each heartbeat and can be felt as a wave of distension in certain arteries where they lie close to the skin (Fig. 16.1). The major pulses are:
- (a) the carotid pulses, one each side of the neck, and
- (b) the femoral pulses, one in each groin.

In addition, a pulse may easily be felt at the wrist, close to the base of the thumb. This is the **radial** pulse. The **ulnar** pulse may also be felt, but rather less easily, at the opposite side of the wrist in a similar position.

Both these pulses may be absent, even in health.

When assessing the circulation, it is vital to feel for one of the major pulses described above. If the pulse cannot be felt in a particular site, another major pulse should be sought. This takes only a few seconds.

The heart rate (pulse rate)

In Chapter 9 (The Heart and Circulation), we noted that the heart rate is typically 60–80 beats per minute in an adult. It is slower in many athletes and faster in babies and children. The heart rate increases with exercise (to meet the increased demands of active muscle for oxygen, the blood flow must increase), fever, fear and following blood loss or prolonged fluid depletion.

The **character** of the pulse is important as well as its rate. One should note when taking the pulse:
- (a) if the pulse is regular or irregular,
- (b) if it is of normal strength or weak, and
- (c) the pulse rate (beats per minute).

Haemorrhage

The cells of the body are supplied with oxygen and nutrients via the blood stream. Thus, the blood must be kept circulating in order to maintain that supply. The blood pressure is the 'force' which maintains the circulation of blood.

Major blood loss reduces the blood pressure. Less severe bleeding is compensated for by an increase in the heart rate, and by the diversion of

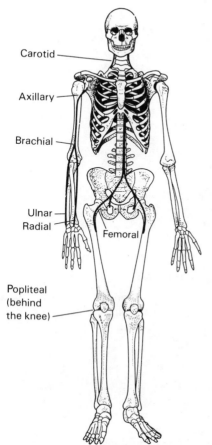

Carotid

Axillary

Brachial

Ulnar
Radial
Femoral

Popliteal
(behind
the knee)

Fig. 16.1 The major pulses.

blood away from the skin and intestine to vital organs, such as the brain. If the blood pressure remains abnormally low for any reason, after a short period of time – even 30 minutes – severe damage will occur to the vital organs, especially the brain, kidneys and heart. The kidneys are particularly sensitive to reduction in their blood flow, and renal failure may follow even short periods of 'shock' (see below).

The body has protective mechanisms to combat haemorrhage. When a blood vessel is cut, the severed ends of the vessel constrict to reduce bleeding (the casualty may even survive a limb being torn off because of this). The constricted vessel reduces blood flow from the damaged ends and allows a clot to form, preventing further blood loss.

Types of bleeding

Arterial. In general, arterial blood is bright red in colour and spurts from the wound in time with the pulse. (The pulmonary artery carries deoxygenated blood from the heart to the lungs. This blood, were one to see it, is darker red.)

Venous. Venous blood is dark red because it is less oxygenated (again, with the exception of the pulmonary veins, which carry oxygenated blood from the lungs to the heart). It tends to well up or gush from a wound but does not spurt.

Capillary. Capillaries are the small vessels linking arteries and veins. Blood oozes from the wound in minor cuts and abrasions. In larger wounds capillary bleeding is overshadowed by arterial and venous bleeding.

Haemorrhage may be classified as:
  (a) **external** or
  (b) **internal**, concealed or revealed (see below).
    Once an assessment of the casualty has been made, priority must be given to arresting major haemorrhage. If haemorrhage is severe, the casualty may require resuscitation. It may not be possible to stop the bleeding completely, but the time gained may keep the casualty alive long enough for him to reach expert help.

Symptoms and signs of major blood loss

1. Evidence of blood loss: **this may be absent.**
2. Pale, cold sweating skin.
3. Restlessness and confusion; altered consciousness.
4. Rapid pulse, weaker than normal.
5. Rapid, shallow respiration (air hunger).
6. Progression to the 'shocked' state (see below).

Treatment of external haemorrhage

1. Apply **direct pressure** over the wound with the hand, or squeeze the edges if it is a cut. If available, use a pad of clean cloth.
2. Lay the casualty flat (horizontal) and elevate the legs; loosen clothing.
3. If the wound is in the arm, elevate this also (elevation reduces the blood pressure in the part and returns blood to vital organs).
4. Tie the pad or dressing in place, preferably with a bandage wrapped several times around. Do not tie it so tightly that a tourniquet is formed. If blood soaks through the dressing, do not remove it but tie more on top.
5. Seek expert help.

Pressure points

If direct pressure does not stop the bleeding (and this is **rare**), the artery to a limb may be compressed where it crosses a bone. This is a 'pressure point' (Fig. 16.2). Remember that such pressure will cut off the blood supply to all the tissue beyond that point (the whole leg in the case of the femoral artery – see Fig. 16.3). Thus, indirect pressure at a pressure point is used as a last resort and **only** if concerted attempts at direct pressure with elevation are unsuccessful.

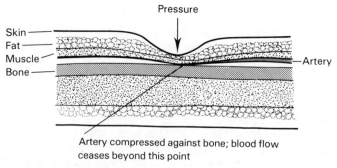

Fig. 16.2 The principle of a pressure point.

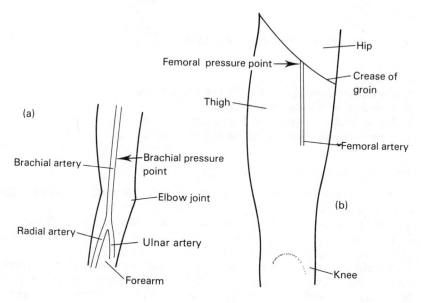

Fig. 16.3a & b Pressure points: (a) brachial; (b) femoral.

Foreign bodies

Do not remove knife blades, pieces of wood, metal or any other foreign body. Make a **ring pad** from a square or triangle of cloth to surround the protruding foreign body (Fig. 16.4). Then apply direct pressure on top of the ring pad.

Internal haemorrhage

The blood loss may be severe **without any external bleeding being visible at all**. This is called **concealed** internal haemorrhage. It may occur following major fractures, for example of the pelvis or limbs, or if the casualty suffers damage to internal organs such as the liver or spleen. Although the blood is not lost to the body as such, **it is lost from the circulation**, with consequent reduction in the blood pressure.

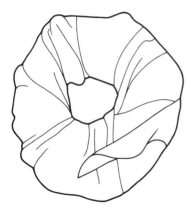

Fig. 16.4 Ring pad.

Even small amounts of blood collecting inside the skull or around the heart may cause major problems, due to pressure on the brain or heart respectively.

Internal haemorrhage may become **revealed** by being lost in the urine, being coughed up or vomited, or simply by the formation of a bruise over the damaged part.

Any shocked patient who has suffered an injury must be assumed to have internal bleeding until proven otherwise.

The marks of seat belts across the chest and abdomen signify severe deceleration. One must constantly bear in mind the possibility of internal bleeding in such patients, and frequent reassessment of the pulse and general condition is necessary.

Treatment

1. Lay the patient down and elevate the legs if possible.
2. Loosen clothing.
3. Cover with one blanket (see below under 'shock').
4. Summon urgent expert help. Make frequent observations of the pulse rate, respiratory rate and conscious level.

Never give patients with major injuries anything by mouth.

CAUSES OF INTERNAL HAEMORRHAGE

Concealed

Fractures – pelvis, long bones, skull.
Damage to organs – liver, spleen, lung, kidney, heart, brain and almost any other.

Revealed

Fractured skull – bleeding from ear or nose.
Direct trauma – to ear, nose, mouth.
Peptic ulcer – dark blood (resembling coffee grounds) vomited.
              – tarry faeces (altered blood).
(N.B. Bright red blood from the rectum is usually due to haemorrhoids.)
Damage to lung or airway – bright red, frothy blood coughed up.
Damage to kidney or bladder – bloodstained urine.
Fractured pelvis with damage to urinary tract (urethra) – **fresh blood** with urine.
Miscarriage or abortion – sudden severe loss of fresh or dark blood from the vagina (N.B. There may be **no** history of a missed period).

Shock states

'Shock' is a term which is often used loosely, resulting in confusion.

In medical terms, 'shock' is the state which results when there is relative or absolute loss of circulating blood volume.

This can be due to many causes, some of which are given below. To visualize the mechanisms producing the shock state, consider Fig. 16.5.

Causes of shock states ('shock')

1. **Loss of circulating volume:**
   (a) haemorrhage;
   (b) prolonged vomiting or diarrhoea – fluid lost replaced from circulation;

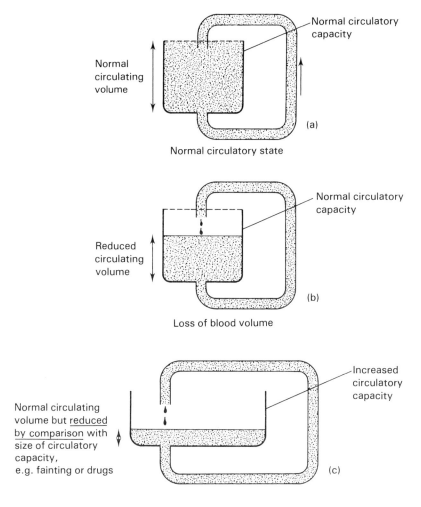

Fig. 16.5 Circulation: (a) normal circulatory state; (b) loss of blood volume; (c) from fainting or drugs.

    (c) burns – due to loss of plasma;
    (d) peritonitis.
2. **Increased circulatory capacity:**
    (a) certain types of fainting attacks;
    (b) severe infections;
    (c) certain drug overdoses;
    (d) pain and fear.

3. **Lack of normal circulation due to 'pump failure':**
   (a) heart attack;
   (b) abnormal heart rhythm (irregular pulse);
   (c) massive pulmonary embolus.

General symptoms and signs of shock states

1. Anxiety; restlessness, progressing to clouding of consciousness and eventual coma.
2. Nausea and vomiting.
3. Pallor and sweating, even though the patient feels cold. (In an attempt to maintain the blood pressure, the blood vessels in the skin constrict. The same part of the nervous system which brings this about, the sympathetic nervous system, supplies the sweat glands.)
4. Fast, weak pulse (but this may be slow or irregular).
5. Rapid, shallow respiration (usually).
Eventually, the heart and respiration may become irregular and then cease.

If no pulse can be felt, or respiration stops, commence resuscitation immediately.

Treatment

1. Lay the patient down and raise the legs. If vomiting occurs, place in the recovery position unless resuscitation is required.
2. Cover with one blanket or a 'space' blanket. Do not warm the patient too much, for example with a hot water bottle, as this may divert blood away from vital organs to the skin.
3. Loosen clothing.
4. Treat any associated injury if possible.
5. Summon expert help.

Do not give anything by mouth. Do not allow smoking.

A conscious casualty's lips can, however, be moistened with a wet tissue.

Fainting

Fainting occurs when the blood supply to the brain is temporarily insufficient. The patient feels dizzy and eventually unconsciousness occurs, and the patient falls to the gound. This in itself should restore the blood supply to the brain and the patient will recover rapidly. Prompt treatment may prevent loss of consciousness.

The cause is usually 'pooling' of blood in the legs due to inactivity, especially in hot environments, or on rising from bed or a warm bath. In this situation there is insufficient blood pressure to maintain circulation to the brain. Certain types of irregular pulse due to heart disease may also make patients prone to fainting.

Symptoms and signs

1. The patient feels dizzy and weak.
2. Pallor.
3. Slow or irregular pulse.

Treatment

1. If unconsciousness has not occurred, sit the patient down and lean him forward with his head on his knees. This brings the head near to the level of the heart and restores blood pressure to the brain. Alternatively, lay the patient flat and raise the legs. This may be more effective.
2. The patient may recover more quickly if placed in a cool environment.
3. **Fully conscious** patients may be allowed sips of water.
4. It may be necessary to treat any injury caused by the patient's fall.

Angina pectoris

This means, literally, pain in the chest. It is now taken to mean pain of cardiac origin which occurs without a coronary artery thrombosis. It is due either to spasm of the coronary arteries (which supply the heart muscle) or because narrowed, diseased arteries cannot supply enough blood to the heart muscle when the heart is working harder, for example with exercise.

The pain is usually only of short duration and is relieved by rest.

Symptoms and signs

1. **Central chest pain**, described as 'heavy', which radiates to the arms (usually the left), jaw, and sometimes the upper abdomen.
2. Pallor and possibly cyanosis.
3. Rapid, shallow respiration. Breathing may be inhibited by the pain.
4. There may be clouding of consciousness.
5. Nausea or vomiting.

Treatment

1. Reassurance.
2. Sit or lie the casualty down. If vomiting has occurred, place in the recovery position.
3. Loosen clothing.

4. If the patient has tablets to take for this condition, allow him to do so. (N.B. Glyceryl trinitrate tablets are allowed to dissolve under the tongue, **not swallowed**).
5. Seek medical advice.

Heart attack (myocardial infarction; coronary thrombosis)

A blood clot may form (thrombosis) in a diseased coronary artery, which causes damage and death of a portion of the heart muscle (myocardial infarction).

Symptoms and signs

1. Sudden onset of severe crushing central chest pain which classically spreads into the left arm but may radiate to the jaw, neck, other arm, abdomen or back.
2. The patient feels faint and may vomit.
3. Pallor, sweating, cyanosis.
4. Rapid, shallow respiration.
5. An irregular pulse may occur.
6. The heart may stop, with sudden collapse of the patient (cardiac arrest).

Treatment

1. IF THERE IS NO PULSE, COMMENCE CARDIOPULMONARY RESUSCITATION IMMEDIATELY.
2. DO NOT GIVE ANYTHING BY MOUTH.
3. If the patient is unconscious, but has a pulse and is breathing, place in the recovery position. **Ensure that the airway is maintained.**
4. **Conscious casualties** should be placed sitting at 45 degrees, and not laid flat. **Do not raise the legs** since this may place a strain on the heart by increasing the return of venous blood.
5. Loosen clothing and reassure the patient.
6. Limit movement as much as possible.
7. Summon medical help immediately.
8. Observe pulse rate, level of consciousness and respiration frequently.

Stroke

There are two types of stroke:
    (a) due to a **cerebral haemorrhage**;
    (b) due to **thrombosis** in a cerebral blood vessel.
    The condition is due to impaired blood supply to, or pressure on, the nerve cells in the brain, which cease to function in the affected area. The

symptoms and signs depend upon which area is damaged. Speech may be affected, and a major stroke may leave the patient paralysed in one or more limbs. Occasionally the airway and swallowing are affected.

Strokes are common in elderly people (over 60) and those with high blood pressure.

Altered consciousness or coma is common.

Symptoms and signs

Any or all of these may occur:
- (a) disorientation;
- (b) difficulty with speech;
- (c) loss of balance;
- (d) weakness or paralysis (saliva may drool from the mouth);
- (e) headache;
- (f) coma;
- (g) incontinence;
- (h) unequal pupils.

Treatment

1. Ensure a clear airway.
2. Reassure the patient. If unconscious, place in the recovery position.
3. Loosen clothing.
4. Summon medical aid.

If pulse or respiration cease, commence resuscitation immediately. Do not give anything by mouth

— 17

The Abdomen

Abdominal pain

Unfortunately, there is a great tendency amongst the public to delay sending for a doctor for pain in the abdomen. Wishful thinking leads the patient to ascribe the trouble to a simple cause such as indigestion; or he may hope that it will soon pass off of its own accord. Failure to call in a doctor promptly for cases of abdominal pain may even lead to death (e.g. from appendicitis), particularly in children.

Many serious conditions cause abdominal pain; these include appendicitis, gastric or duodenal ulcers, peritonitis, intestinal obstruction or inflammation and diseases of other internal organs (such as the gall bladder or kidneys). The character of the pain, the location, severity and duration will help the doctor in his diagnosis. If in addition there is tenderness, increased temperature and pulse rate, diarrhoea or vomiting, the patient must be seen without delay.

Treatment

All cases of sudden abdominal pain should be treated by putting the patient to bed and sending for a doctor. The patient should be allowed to adopt a comfortable position (this is often sitting up).

Hernia (rupture)

A hernia consists of the protrusion of some of the contents of the abdomen through a weakness in the abdominal wall. It takes the form of a swelling under the skin (usually situated in the groin) and is aggravated by recurrent strain, for example coughing, the repeated lifting of heavy objects or a weak abdominal wall.

A hernia by itself does not require first aid treatment, but it is liable to serious complications. If there is intense pain, and if the swelling becomes firm and tender this is a dangerous event. If the intestine in the hernia does not return to the abdomen a bowel obstruction may ensue; if the blood supply of the intestine is constricted by the pressure, strangulation of the intestine will follow.

Treatment

A doctor should be sent for quickly, because it is sometimes possible to avoid an immediate operation by replacing the hernia. On no account, however, should the first aider attempt this process himself, as it is both dangerous and difficult.

The patient should be put to bed and advised to lie on his back with his knees bent and his head and shoulders raised. This position relieves the tension of the muscles around the hernia. In addition, the foot of the bed should be raised. Nothing should be given by mouth.

Renal colic

After periods of hot weather combined with excessive sweating and exercise, particularly if the patient has not been drinking a lot of fluid, small stones may form in the kidney. These pass down to the bladder causing severe pains. This pain passes from the loin to the pubis and comes in severe spasms. It may be so severe that the patient writhes on the floor and vomits. There may be an urge to pass urine and there may be some blood in the urine. The patient will require assessment and investigation, so should be taken to a doctor.

Acute urinary retention

This condition is common in elderly men. The history is of increasing difficulty in passing urine; the patient gets up at night, dribbles urine and has difficulty in starting and stopping passing urine. After a period of this disability he occasionally is unable to pass urine: acute retention. He wants to pass urine but because of the pressure of the prostate is not able to do so. There is increasing lower abdominal pain with inability to pass urine and the bladder is distended.

The patient, if the lesion is long-standing, may be uraemic with increasing drowsiness and a foul-smelling breath. This condition is an acute emergency and the patient should be seen by a doctor or taken to hospital urgently.

Closed abdominal injury

Injuries to the liver, spleen, kidneys or gut in the abdomen are becoming more common with high speed road traffic accidents. Wearing a seat belt protects most from injury, but with high speeds severe bruising of the abdomen and chest can occur, and sometimes there will be internal injury.

Symptoms and signs

1. The patient will complain of pain on moving or breathing.
2. On examination, there may be bruising of the abdomen. If this is seen it shows the blow was severe.
3. On palpation, tenderness and hardness of the muscles is found.
4. The signs of shock will develop, so observation of the patient's face, pulse, level of consciousness and general condition should be made frequently.

Treatment

The patient must be moved to hospital if intra-abdominal injury is suspected. Oral fluids or solids must NOT be given. The patient should lie down on a stretcher. A pillow under the knees will give some comfort. If there is an associated injury to the chest, the patient would be more comfortable and find breathing easier if placed semi-recumbent.

Open abdominal injury

Open wounds of the abdominal wall may be either simple or accompanied by protrusion of the intestines.

Treatment

The patient should be placed in such a position that the edges of the wound come together, and a dry temporary dressing applied. Only if the wound is obviously superficial should the first aider use the routine treatment of cleaning and dressing, e.g. when there is no danger of anything passing into the abdominal cavity.

Where there is protrusion of the intestine the patient should be laid on his back with shoulders raised and knees bent. Avoid handling the gut as much as possible. The abdominal organs which are visible should be covered with hot flannels soaked in salt solution (1 teaspoon to the pint, appx. ½ litre). Excess solution should be wrung out of the cloths, which should be as hot as the first aider can comfortably handle. The saline keeps the exposed intestine warm and moist and the dressing should be covered if possible with a plastic bag. Treatment for shock and emotional distress will also be needed.

Swallowed foreign body

Children are at most risk. Coins, buttons, beads, pins and stones are all commonly swallowed. Most pass through the gut without causing damage, but a sharp object such as a pin or kirbigrip may perforate the bowel.

Symptoms and signs may be minor, but abdominal pain may occur if the bowel is perforated. The diagnosis is usually made from the history.

Treatment

1. Do not allow anything by mouth.
2. Seek medical aid.

Foreign bodies in the vagina or rectum

Sharp objects may penetrate the abdomen with serious consequences. Blunt objects may cause bleeding and discharge if present for a long time.

Treatment

Seek medical attention.

— 18

Wounds and their Treatment

WOUNDS

A wound is a break in continuity; this occurs frequently in the skin or the mucous membranes. Often internal organs such as the heart, lung or kidney will suffer from wounds due to various forms of trauma.

In any wound, when blood vessels are damaged, the cut or torn ends contract to reduce bleeding. Torn vessels do this better than cleanly cut ones. Eventually a clot forms, which stops further bleeding. If there has been loss of tissue, new connective tissue and blood vessels grow in to fill the gap, but healing takes longer than in a cleanly-cut wound. Scars are the result of this growth of connective tissue.

Types of wounds

Incised wound. This is a straightforward cut with clean edges, such as that produced by a knife. They are often deep, and tend to gape. Arteries may be cut, resulting in profuse bleeding.

When closed they heal quickly leaving a fine scar. This is healing by first intention.

Laceration. The wound edges are torn rather than cut. The edges are irregular and bruised. Examples are wounds produced by barbed wire, ragged metal edges or shearing forces when a limb is trapped in machinery. Bleeding may be less than in incised wounds because the torn blood vessels contract more effectively. Gunshot wounds and machinery accidents cause severe lacerations which may involve the underlying muscle. A graze is a very superficial laceration, and if not infected will heal with minimum scarring. Lacerated wounds heal slowly and can leave unpleasant scars. The edges are often excised by the doctor before stitching to leave a straight scar.

Puncture wounds. These may vary in depth and severity according to the cause. Simple punctures which occur from standing on a nail or piece of glass rarely produce much bleeding. The danger in these lies in subsequent infection, especially if a piece of material (foreign body) has been left inside.

Bites from dogs, cats and humans are nearly always infected. **Tetanus** is the worst consequence of deep contamination with soil, manure and foreign bodies.

More serious puncture wounds occur from stabbing (accidental or otherwise) with knives, railings, wooden stakes etc. Such wounds may result in serious damage to deep blood vessels, nerves or internal organs. There may be profuse internal haemorrhage and shock. Infection may develop if the implement was not clean, or if pieces of clothing have been carried into the wound. Penetrating objects should be left in the patient to be removed at the hospital. Any bleeding can then be dealt with immediately by the surgeon.

Contusion. A contusion is simply a 'bruise' which results from bleeding under the skin. It should be remembered in such cases that deeper structures may have been damaged, muscle is frequently torn and there may be a fracture.

Burns. See Chapter 30.

War wounds. See below.

Traumatic amputation. Some injuries may result in a limb or digit being torn or cut off. The body's natural response to injury by contraction of the blood vessels may prevent serious haemorrhage (casualties have been known to crawl great distances to get help). The wound should be treated by direct pressure with a pad on the stump to control bleeding. Recent developments in microsurgical techniques have made reattachment of amputated limbs a possibility. Time is of the essence, however, and the amputated part should be placed in a plastic bag to prevent it drying out and to minimize further damage. This is placed in another bag containing ice. The ambulance service should be told there has been an amputation so that as much warning as possible can be given to the receiving hospital.

First aid measures for wounds

Small wounds should always be washed and covered with a sterile dressing. Larger ones, especially if they could be contaminated, should be seen by a doctor. For **any** infected wound the patient should be strongly advised to seek medical advice. Any patient who has not been immunized against tetanus should seek medical attention **even if the wound is apparently trivial** and in **every** case if it is a puncture wound. If an infection seems to be spreading, the patient feels generally unwell, has a fever or becomes shocked, urgent medical advice must be sought as the risk of septicaemia or distant spread of the organism is very real.

Foreign bodies embedded in a wound

Fragments of metal, wood, glass etc. are commonly found embedded in wounds.

Treatment

Attempts to remove small foreign bodies by washing off with water are often unsuccessful. Larger pieces should not be removed, as further damage may result. Instead, place dressings around the foreign body and make a ring pad (Fig. 16.4) to surround the fragment and allow pressure to be applied to the wound but not the fragment. Alternatively, 'sausages' of cotton wool may be used. Cover all this with more dressings and bandage in place.

Never apply direct pressure over the foreign body itself

If severe bleeding has occurred, apply pressure to the edges of the wound until a ring pad and bandage can be applied.

Transfixion injuries

These may occur if, for example, the casualty is impaled on railings or fencing.

Treatment

1. **DO NOT** attempt removal under any circumstances.
2. If the casualty is conscious, support him so that he is not suspended on the impaling item. Reassure strongly and gain his confidence.
3. Treat all visible injuries as adequately as possible without moving the patient.
4. Send a bystander to call for an ambulance **and the fire service**, stating what has happened (specialized cutting apparatus may be required to free the casualty).

Splinters

Wood and metal splinters in the skin, or underneath the nails, are an everyday occurrence. There is usually a history of sudden pain or pricking.

Treatment

1. Attempt to wash the splinter away.
2. If this fails, try to grasp the splinter with forceps (tweezers), but do not injure the skin further.
3. If 2 is unsuccessful, seek medical attention.

Remember, a splinter constitutes a puncture wound. The patient may be at risk from tetanus if unimmunized.

Fish hooks and wire

The point of a fish hook or sharp wire can simply be removed by gently pulling it out. The area should then be washed well with soap and water. If the barb of a fish hook is embedded as well, push the hook through in order to cut off the barb.

The risk of tetanus from such a wound is a very real one.

Treatment

Such injuries are best treated as for embedded foreign bodies (see above) and medical attention sought as soon as possible.

GENERAL PRINCIPLES OF TREATMENT

There are four principal objects in the treatment of wounds.
1. To arrest haemorrhage.
2. To treat shock.
3. To prevent sepsis.
4. To promote healing.
These are of equal importance, and should be treated in the order named.

Extent of treatment

The amount of treatment supplied in any particular case depends on the facilities that are available and the environment of the accident. In street accidents, for example, severe bleeding must be stopped immediately and then treatment for shock begun; but the wound itself should only be treated by quick and temporary methods, more thorough treatment being postponed until the patient has been removed to a suitable centre. Similarly, when several casualties have occurred as a result of a single accident, the extent of treatment must be limited.

There are two methods of treating wounds, routine and temporary.

Routine method

This is the best method of treating a wound, but can only be undertaken when circumstances are favourable, e.g. when there is a satisfactory first aid room available. The routine method should be used in the following cases:

1. For all minor wounds, e.g. cuts, scratches, abrasions etc., which are unlikely to require the services of a doctor.
2. For small wounds which will ultimately require medical treatment, but when there is no need for hurry; the method is then undertaken as a preparation for the doctor.
3. For larger wounds, when the first aider is working under the instructions of a doctor.
4. For large wounds when it is unlikely that medical facilities will be obtainable for at least six hours. In this case, the routine method should be postponed until the patient has been adequately treated for shock.

Temporary methods

These are emergency treatments which can be undertaken for all accidents which occur under unfavourable conditions, e.g. in the street. The methods must be altered slightly according to the probable length of time which will elapse before medical services become available.

Routine treatment

Haemorrhage. When it is obvious that severe bleeding is taking place, the first aider must not waste time with refinements but must at once take steps to control the bleeding.

Position. The patient should be placed in a suitable position for treatment. Blood escapes with less force when the patient is lying down, and for this reason, in cases of severe wounds, he should be made to lie flat; in less serious cases, when there is only slight haemorrhage, he may be allowed to sit up.

Patient care. Immediate preventive treatment for anxiety and shock should be adopted. The importance of sympathetic encouragement and reassurance cannot be too greatly stressed.

Exposure of wound. The wound should now be partially exposed by cutting away clothing where necessary and removing boots, etc. While doing this, the first aider will gain some idea of the severity of the bleeding.

   If blood is pouring through the clothing haemorrhage is severe, and no time should be wasted in taking immediate steps to control it. When, however, as is often the case, partial exposure of the wound discloses that the bleeding is not so bad as was anticipated, the first aider may leave a small piece of clothing still covering the wound; this will act as a temporary protection against the entrance of germs while he is making preparations for actual treatment.

Cleanliness. While removing the clothing, especially boots, the first aider is sure to dirty his fingers. He should wash his hands thoroughly with soap and water.

Prepare apparatus. All apparatus required for the treatment of the wound should now be prepared and placed by the side of the patient, spread out on a clean towel. Appliances will include bowls, antiseptics, warm water, dressings, scissors and forceps. (Forceps are required for handling dressings.)

Bowls and instruments should be sterilized before use, by allowing them to simmer in water in a clean saucepan for a few minutes; alternatively, they may be flamed – a method of quick sterilization which consists of pouring a small quantity of methylated spirit into a bowl and then lighting it, when the heat produced will be sufficient to destroy any germs that are present. Instruments can similarly be flamed in an emergency to save time, although the process is liable to damage the metal of which they are made.

Cleanliness. The first aider will do well to wash his hands again at this stage. The importance of cleanliness cannot be overestimated. No matter how clean the hands may appear, it is probable that numerous germs exist on the fingers which, if allowed to come into contact with the wound, will increase the risk of sepsis.

Complete exposure. The wound may now be completely exposed, and should be examined to determine its variety, the type of haemorrhage that is occurring, and the possible presence of foreign bodies. The risk of cut tendons must be borne in mind.

If there is no fracture, raise the injured part and support it in an elevated position in order to reduce haemorrhage.

Foreign bodies. Foreign bodies lying loose in the depths of the wound may now be removed, but it is inadvisable to remove those which appear to be deeply imbedded, for fear of precipitating further haemorrhage. Occasionally, for example, a piece of glass will perforate a blood-vessel, but will remain in the wound like a cork, preventing the escape of blood. If the foreign body is removed at this stage, severe bleeding may result. The first aider must not search for foreign bodies by probing the wound, this procedure should only be undertaken by a doctor.

Cleansing the wound. The wound should now be thoroughly cleansed with a suitable antiseptic solution. Great care must be taken to avoid contaminating the wound with dirt derived from the skin. For this reason, a wound should always be cleansed from within outwards and a number of swabs used, each one being thrown away directly it has touched the surrounding skin. Small pieces of cotton wool, well soaked in antiseptic, should be dabbed over the surface, or squeezed so that the antiseptic penetrates to the depths of the wound. Cleanse the skin around with fresh swabs.

As regards the solution to be employed for this cleansing, many suitable antiseptics are available. Thus, hydrogen peroxide (10 volumes) diluted with an equal quantity of water is an excellent preparation, but its disadvantage is that it does not preserve its strength once a bottle has been opened, unless kept in a dark bottle and stored in a dark place. Many proprietary antiseptics, such as Dettol and Cetavlon, and antiseptics containing chlorhexidine and povidone iodine are also satisfactory; the solution employed, however, should always be weak (e.g. 1 in 20 Dettol), because the chief value of bathing the wound is merely mechanical and is an attempt to wash away dirt and germs. Strong antiseptics may cause harmful effects on the tissues.

Bathing should be continued for some time, depending on the size of the wound and the degree of contamination. Five to ten minutes' cleansing of a wound, in this manner, may go far in preventing sepsis. Alternatively the wound may be washed under a running tap or jet.

Further examination. During the process of bathing the wound, the first aider should make the important decision as to whether a doctor's services are necessary, either to deal with bleeding or to insert stitches.

If a wound gapes at all, and still more if fat is visible under the skin, it will require stitching. When after thorough bathing a decision is made that stitching is desirable, the wound should be covered with a temporary dressing and all subsequent treatment left to the doctor. In cases of doubt it is always advisable to obtain a medical opinion, for wounds heal much more quickly when stitched and the risk of sepsis is thereby reduced.

Application of antiseptic. When a wound is trivial, or if it is unlikely that a doctor can be obtained for some hours, the wound and the skin around it should be painted with a weak antiseptic; suitable antiseptics are Dettol, TCP, and those containing chlorhexidine and povidone iodine.

Dressing. A suitable dressing should now be applied. This usually consists of several thicknesses of gauze.

Dry dressings are usually used, because they are readily available and encourage healing; but when a wound looks dirty in spite of cleansing and is liable to become septic, an antibiotic cream or powder should be used.

A good pad of cotton wool should then be put over the dressing and tied firmly in position by a narrow bandage.

It will be appreciated that a pad tied firmly in position is intended to stop the bleeding. Care must be taken, however, not to bandage too tightly in cases of fractures or when foreign bodies are present in the wound, owing to the risk of producing complications. Whenever possible prepared sterile dressings should be used.

Support. Suitable support should be supplied to the affected part, and, in severe wounds involving limbs, it is desirable to use a splint to relieve pain and reduce the risks of secondary shock.

Medical aid. Arrangements should now be made for a medical opinion, since injections of preventive drugs may be desirable to avoid the risk of tetanus and other complications.

Temporary treatments

When medical facilities, e.g. a hospital or dressing station, are near at hand, it is only necessary to cover a wound temporarily with a standard pad-and-bandage dressing. Haemorrhage must, of course, be arrested, and it is an advantage to cleanse the skin round the wound with surgical spirit or other suitable antiseptic if available.

However, when there is no opportunity of obtaining medical aid for several hours and there is no chance of removing the patient to a suitable centre, the wound should be covered with a dressing using a dilute antiseptic solution after cleaning.

It will be understood that temporary methods are only modifications of the routine treatment already described.

War wounds

Wounds caused by bullets and the fragments of shells and bombs, etc., may be of any variety and are frequently accompanied by complications. Unpleasant injuries occur in urban terrorism, with bomb explosions causing blast injuries. Thus a limb may be severed completely, leaving a large exposed stump, while any part of the body may be severely crushed by falling masonry or debris.

A characteristic feature of war injuries is that they are often multiple, i.e. a patient may sustain a number of wounds simultaneously.

The lacerated wounds which occur in warfare may be very extensive and are often associated with damage to underlying muscles, which may be bruised or torn and hence ooze blood freely. Marked shock is usually present; this is due to loss of blood, muscle damage and fractures.

Many war wounds are of the puncture variety. In this case, the missile enters the skin and passes along a track to a considerable depth; it may finally lodge in an internal organ or even leave the body through another wound.

The wound of entrance, or point of entry, may be very small and appear like a small, punched-out hole, the edges of which may be turned inwards and burnt.

The track may follow any direction, and during its course through the body the missile may damage important organs, causing internal injuries;

thus, bones may be shattered, nerves and blood-vessels severed, and, if the wound involves the trunk, organs such as the intestines and lungs may be perforated.

The wound (point) of exit, if present, is generally larger than that of entry; its edges may appear turned outwards and torn. It will be appreciated that if there is no point of exit, the missile has been retained within the body.

The puncture wounds sustained in warfare may be very deceptive, because all the first aider may notice is a small superficial injury of no apparent consequence. Yet this may be the point of entry of a severe puncture wound and serious damage may be present within the body. Moreover, since wounds of this type are often multiple, a small entry wound may entirely escape notice unless a thorough examination of every inch of the body is undertaken; this, however, involves completely undressing the patient and is not justifiable at the scene of incident owing to the risk of exposure which increases shock. Hence the supreme importance of quickly removing such casualties to a hospital or first aid post, where a complete examination can be performed by a doctor under suitable conditions.

So far as the treatment of war wounds is concerned, the first aider must proceed according to general principles, adopting quick and temporary methods so that his patient can be speedily removed to shelter. The wounds should be covered with suitable first dressings and haemorrhage arrested. If one pad is not sufficient, apply another pad and bandage on top and bandage firmly. Fractures should be controlled after ensuring that the airway is clear.

— 19

Wound Infections

A healing wound is always inflamed due to the increased blood supply to the area while the tissue is being repaired. Infection with microorganisms, usually bacteria, results in proliferation of the white cells of the blood to combat the infection. Dead white cells, bacteria and tissue debris form 'pus', which accumulates in infected wounds. Medical attention must always be sought for infected wounds, however trivial they may seem.

We must define the term 'infection'. All newborn animals are quickly invaded by bacteria and viruses. Thus, in a newborn baby the bowel contents are sterile, but within hours organisms come to inhabit the intestine. The same occurs in the mouth and on the skin. Certain parts of the body, however, remain sterile, such as the urinary tract, middle and inner ear.

Organisms can regularly be grown from such sites as the skin or gut **but they do not produce any disease**. Such organisms are part of the 'normal flora'. They help to prevent the establishment of disease-producing (pathogenic) organisms and may thus be regarded as protective. When a tissue or organ is colonized by bacteria or viruses which are not normally found there, interference with normal function may occur and infection is said to be present.

Occasionally, antibiotic treatment may interfere with the balance of the normal flora, as can changes in the acidity of secretions on the skin or in the genitourinary tract. Some organisms are part of the normal flora in certain sites, but when they become established in another site (for example, 'gut organisms' in the urinary tract), they become pathogenic. Blood borne infection (septicaemia) may lead to 'septic shock' with low blood pressure and poor peripheral blood flow. Such patients are critically ill.

Routes of entry to the body

Via the skin

The skin provides a good barrier against infection. Sweat contains substances which inhibit bacterial growth and the growth of the normal flora tends to swamp any pathogenic bacteria. Occasionally, however, hair follicles and small wounds may become infected. Especially dangerous are puncture wounds (see above) which may allow the spores of the tetanus organism to germinate in a favourable environment.

Tetanus is a disease of the nervous system manifested by stiffness of the muscles (particularly those of the jaw, hence the popular name of 'lock jaw') and eventual respiratory weakness and death from respiratory insufficiency.

The disease is caused by a toxin produced by the organism *Clostridium tetani*, which affects nerve cells. Spores of this organism are present in soil, animal faeces and household dust. They are very resistant and remain viable for a very long time. They germinate in conditions where there is little oxygen, such as a deep puncture wound. Only when the spores have germinated is the toxin produced.

Tetanus is often a fatal disease if untreated, but is very easily prevented by immunization with a chemically modified form of the toxin called *tetanus toxoid*. A course of three injections is required, followed by booster doses every five years.

Via mucous membranes

The 'skin' which lines the mouth, respiratory tract, gut and genitourinary tract is known as the mucous membrane. Many viruses, as well as such organisms as syphilis, gain entry this way. Coughing and sneezing following infection with, for example, respiratory viruses, produces clouds of infected droplets which are then inhaled by others. Influenza, the common cold, diphtheria and tuberculosis are all spread in this way.

Burns

A burned area loses its natural skin barrier, and the protective exudate which forms over the burn wound is an ideal place for bacteria to grow. Large burns very easily become infected. Patients may die of overwhelming infection rather than from the burn wound itself.

Direct injection

The infectious organism may be injected into the body by an insect bite (malaria), an animal bite (rabies), or on some object making a puncture wound or in transfused blood or plasma (hepatitis). Hepatitis is spread between drug addicts in this way, as they often share and reuse the same syringes and needles.

Epidemics

Most cases of bacterial infection occur occasionally as isolated events (sporadic). Sometimes, however, many cases occur together. This is especially true of viral infections, but also applies to some bacterial cases, especially food poisoning. Such related events occurring together constitute an epidemic.

The body's response to infection

Localized infections

If the infection is localized, e.g. in a small wound, the body attempts to prevent its spread by pouring in white blood cells, which attack the offending organism. The response is enhanced if the body has encountered the organism before. In addition, certain white cells produce chemical substances called **antibodies**, which are specific to the infecting organism. They are able to activate certain chemicals in the plasma which damage the foreign cells. Other types of white cell then engulf the damaged cells and cell debris and remove them from the body.

Inflammation is associated with this process, as the blood vessels become more permeable to white cells and fluid. Such infected sites are hot, red and tender to the touch. Pus may be visible under the skin, or may be localized into an abscess, which may eventually burst.

Generalized infection

When spread has occurred beyond the site of infection the situation has become very serious indeed, and distant sites, such as the brain or bone, may become infected. Certain organisms may release toxins into the blood which cause collapse and the development of septic shock. This condition may be fatal if not rapidly treated.

20

Fractures

A fracture is a break in continuity of a bone; this may vary from a crack to a complete break (Fig. 20.1).

Causes

Fractures result from the application of force to the skeleton. The force may originate outside the body and may be direct or indirect.

Direct force: the fracture is usually straight across the bone, which breaks at the site of impact.

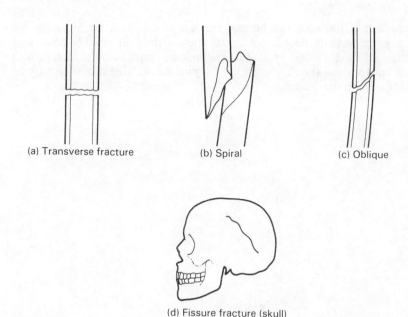

(a) Transverse fracture   (b) Spiral   (c) Oblique

(d) Fissure fracture (skull)

Fig. 20.1 Fractures: (a) transverse; (b) spiral; (c) oblique; (d) fissure fracture (skull).

Indirect force: this usually results in a spiral fracture, the cause being force applied from a distance, e.g. a fall on the arm may cause forced violent rotation of the bones, resulting in spiral fractures. Muscular action may cause fractures by forcible contraction (for example, ribs may be broken by coughing).

Types

Fissure fractures

Fissure fractures are 'crack' fractures and may result from direct or indirect force.

Oblique fractures

Oblique fractures result from a combination of direct and indirect force.

Closed fractures

In closed fractures (see Figs. 20.2, 20.3 and 20.4) the bone has been broken but the overlying skin is intact. There is always damage to the adjacent muscles and blood vessels, so a collection of blood, the fracture haematoma, is always present.

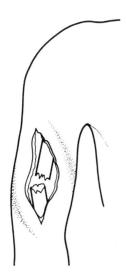

Fig. 20.2 Open fracture of humerus. Note the large skin wound leading down to the fracture.

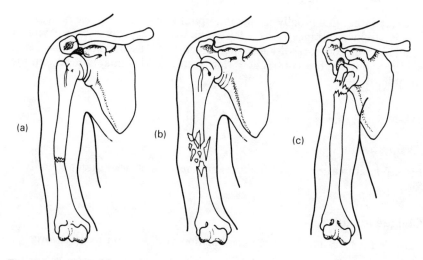

Fig. 20.3 Varieties of fracture: (a) closed; (b) comminuted; (c) accompanied by dislocation.

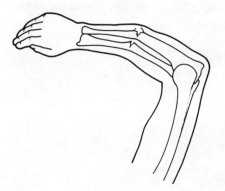

Fig. 20.4 Greenstick fracture of radius and ulna.

Greenstick fractures

Children's bones are much softer than those of adults, and when force is applied to them they tend to bend and split like a green branch of a young tree (rather than breaking straight across as in the adult). The thick periosteum holds the ends of the bone together. Greensticks are generally closed fractures, but occasionally with external wounds they become open.

Open fractures

In open fractures there is a break in the skin or mucous membrane overlying the fracture. There are four common types of open or compound fractures:
1. Open from without, i.e. the wound on the skin surface leads directly to the fracture site (e.g. a gunshot or hatchet wound).
2. Open from within, i.e. a sharp end of the bone penetrates the skin or membrane. This is usually smaller and less dangerous.
3. Fractures of the skull may involve an air sinus or the middle ear, which bleeds through the torn eardrum.
4. Broken ribs may penetrate the underlying lung.
   Note: open fractures are dangerous because of the risk of infection. Bacteria can invade the wound and infect the ends of the bone. External wounds may carry strands of contaminated clothing or dirt into the bone. Fractures of the skull involving the frontal sinus are liable to infect the membranes covering the brain causing meningitis.

Complicated fractures

These occur when the jagged ends of the bone fragments damage blood vessels, nerves or a joint. Broken bones in the trunk may penetrate the lung, heart or liver. In fractures of the skull the brain is usually damaged.

Depressed fractures

These occur in the skull when the broken ends of the bones are pressed inwards. This is a form of complicated fracture.

Comminuted fractures

In these cases, the bone is broken into several fragments. This is serious because there will be more muscle damage with more bleeding at the fracture site. In the tibia and femur, several pints of blood may gather around the fracture.

Impacted fractures

After a heavy fall, the fracture may be impacted by the force. This is often seen at the upper end of the humerus. The nature of these fractures makes them stable and the bone ends do not move.

Combinations of these types of fracture often occur, and an open fracture may be both comminuted and complicated. Greenstick and impacted fractures are generally closed. Without x-rays it is not easy to diagnose comminuted, greenstick, impacted or depressed fractures.

Pathological fractures

These occur when the bone is weakened by loss of calcium, infection or cancer. Minimal force will cause a break in such cases. In old age the bones are more brittle, and may break spontaneously due to calcium loss, which is part of the ageing process. This kind of fracture is often seen in the body of a vertebra or the neck of the femur.

Stress fractures

Stress caused by repeated minor trauma, as in athletic training, can cause small cracks in the cortex of the bone. These are hard to diagnose and must be suspected in those involved in strenuous training, such as jogging or marathon running, when the bone is painful and there is localized tenderness after repeated prolonged activity.

Methods of diagnosis

It is important when making a diagnosis of a fracture (see Fig. 20.5) to
   (a)   have a history of the accident,
   (b)   fully understand what the patient is complaining of, and
   (c)   carry out a physical examination of the site of the suspected fracture.

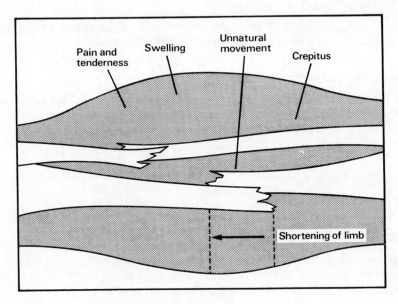

Fig. 20.5 The physical signs and symptoms of a fracture.

History

The patient will generally be able to say what happened, or there may be a witness to the accident.

Symptoms

The patient will describe what he feels, complaining of severe pain, loss of use of the limb and may even say he has heard or felt a crack. It is very important to listen carefully to the description as there will always be something significant to be learned.

Signs: examining a suspected fracture

Deformity. A change in the normal limb contour may be obvious when compared with the opposing one. Angulation of the fracture may be seen.

Irregularity. During a gentle examination of the bone with the fingertips it may feel irregular, e.g. there may be an area of sharpness or a bump may be felt.

Shortening. This is mainly seen in leg fractures. One leg may be obviously shorter than the other. Sometimes a tape measure may be required.

Swelling. After a fracture there is oedema and bleeding from the small blood vessels under the skin and from damaged muscles. The swelling increases and may continue for up to forty-eight hours. Bruising will become obvious, but blood may track for some distance under the skin from the point of impact; thus the bruise may appear quite a distance away from the site of the fracture.

Tenderness. The bone will feel tender, and this is strongly suggestive of fracture. In stress or impacted fractures this may be the only positive sign. Very gentle fingertip pressure will ascertain it.

Crepitus. This peculiar grating sensation may be reported by the patient. Sometimes it is felt when he moves accidentally. It should not be tested for.

Unnatural movement. This may be seen when patients attempt to move a limb and the bone moves at the fracture, not the joint.

The diagnosis

Tenderness over a bone must be regarded as indicative of a fracture until proved otherwise. This cardinal sign is always present. Many of the signs mentioned above may not be seen or may not be obvious. The combination, however, of two or three signs and symptoms should be treated as evidence of a fracture. If the patient is in shock with severe pain in the limb, this should be treated as a fracture and requires urgent investigation.

Principles of first aid treatment

1. Open fractures require dressing urgently to stop bleeding and prevent further infection of the wound.
2. Bone fragments should be splinted to prevent movement. This minimizes the possibility of shock or complications, or a closed fracture becoming an open one.
3. The patient should be moved to a doctor or hospital after first aid.

Prevention of movement

Support. The patient will often hold the affected limb himself. The first aider should take a firm grip of the limb above and below the fracture, thus supporting the limb and preventing movement.

Slings. When applying body bandages, the upper limbs are often supported with arm slings first.

Splints. These are often used but they need padding and careful application, particularly if the patient has to travel far.

Body splints. This is the simplest method of immobilization. With careful application of bandages the uninjured part of the body is used to splint the fractured limb (Fig. 20.6).

Rules for body splinting.
1. Bandages must never encircle the limb at the fracture site. They must always be applied above and below the fracture because the fracture site always swells, and if it is constricted by bandages complications are possible.
2. The bandage above the fracture is always tied before the bandage below: by doing this the limb can be placed in the correct position.
3. Padding is necessary between the injury and the part acting as support, to assist in immobilization.
4. Bandages must be firm to prevent further movement of the bone fragments, but not so tight as to endanger the circulation. It is important to remember that swelling will continue.
5. Bandages should be tied without undue disturbance of the patient. If a bandage can be passed under the limb using a stick to push the bandage

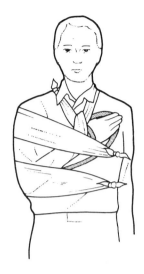

Fig. 20.6 Example of body splint.

through, this will save too much movement. The hollows of the body – the small of the back, the backs of the knees and ankles – can be utilized for this purpose. The bandages can then be gently worked to the desired location.

6. Body splinting must be gently done in an unhurried manner so that the fracture is not moved and the patient does not suffer.

7. Bandages should be checked often and the circulation through the limb observed while the patient is being moved to medical aid. In this way complications are avoided. If the circulation is poor the bandages must be loosened.

Points on method of treatment

When the injured limb is seen to be twisted, displaced or lies under the body, gentle pulling (traction) is permitted. The limb can be gently straightened and this will improve circulation. This manoeuvre enables splintage to be applied easily and effectively.

Observation

This must be repeated frequently. The pulse should be watched beyond the fracture: the circulation in the nail beds of the fingers or toenails should be observed regularly, and compared with the first aider's own. Dusky blue or a whitish hue suggests the bandages are too tight and need to be relaxed.

Healing of fractures

The natural process of union in a fracture enables the broken bone to heal without causing permanent disability, providing the fracture is kept in good alignment and is immobilized properly. A fracture haematoma develops between the disrupted ends of the bones. This clots and, with the surrounding swelling of the muscles, causes a tender swollen area. New cells and small blood vessels grow into this clot, which then forms granulation tissue. Bone-producing cells from the periosteum (the membrane covering the bone) move into the growing tissue and 'woven bone callus' starts to appear about 10 days after the fracture. This forms a firm support to hold the fragments together (Fig. 20.7).

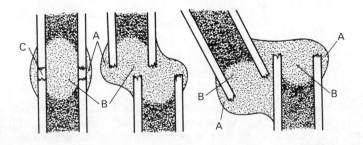

Fig. 20.7 Healing of fractures: (a) outer callus; (b) inner callus; (c) permanent callus. Note: of the three fractures shown, two are healing in a poor position.

If the bone is properly splinted this support is reinforced by permanent callus growing between the fragments and consolidating to hard bone. This is the final bony union. After this the outer and inner lines of callus gradually disappear in the process of remodelling. In children particularly, it is often impossible to know where the fracture was.

FRACTURES OF THE UPPER LIMB

Fractured clavicle

The weight of the upper limb is carried through the clavicle to the sternum and the arm is suspended by many strong muscles attached to this bone. It is commonly fractured in sporting activities, frequently by indirect force and occasionally by direct injury (Fig. 20.8).

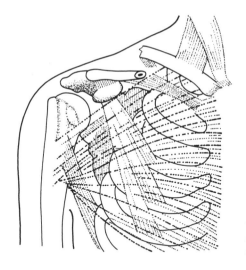

Fig. 20.8 Fracture of clavicle. Note displacement and overlap of fragments and the attached muscles.

Diagnosis

History. Usually the patient falls forward onto the arm and puts out his hand to break his fall. The full weight of the body is then thrown onto the arm.

Symptoms. He describes the pain occurring in the region of the clavicle, and his arm becoming useless.

Signs. On examination he is seen standing supporting the weight of the arm, as this tends to pull the outer fragment down. He is obviously in pain and may be winded by the effect of the fall. It is easy to compare the bone with that of the other side; the deformity, swelling and tenderness will be obvious and, indeed, the end of the fracture is easily felt. Penetration of the skin by the proximal fragment occasionally occurs. This, of course, would be an open injury.

Treatment

This is directed towards supporting the weight of the limb and stabilizing it.
1. It is best done by the use of a **triangular sling**. This is applied after removing the coat, always remembering to take the good arm out of the jacket first. The weight of the arm should be supported by an assistant whilst the triangular sling is being applied. This should take the weight across the other shoulder. The arm is then secured to the side of the chest with a **broad bandage** (Fig. 20.9). After this the pulse should be checked.

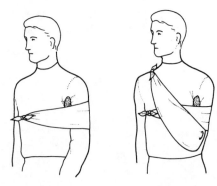

Fig. 20.9 Treatment for fractured clavicle (standard method).

2. Alternatively, the **three-ring** bandage should be applied. Two narrow bandages are tied round each shoulder, padding being applied underneath that on the injured shoulder particularly. A third bandage is then tied on the back between the two rings and is tightened to make the arm secure and comfortable. Additional comfort may then be obtained by applying a triangular sling to support the weight (Fig. 20.10). At all stages the pulse at the wrist should be checked.

Fractures of the scapula

History. Fractures of the scapula may occur by indirect force transmitted in a fall, with a fracture through the glenoid or neck, or by direct force across the blade of the scapula when it may be associated with fractures of the ribs.

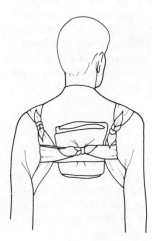

Fig. 20.10 Treatment of fracture of one or both clavicles (three-bandage method).

Symptoms. The patient complains of pain and inability to lift the arm.

Signs. On examination there is swelling at the shoulder joint and inability to move the arm. The patient usually will be supporting the weight of his arm with the other arm.

Treatment. A good, firm triangular sling is necessary to take the weight of the arm, and the arm can be further stabilized by applying a broad bandage around the upper arm. The circulation at the wrist should be checked frequently. If this is interfered with, it may be necessary to remove the broad bandage.

Fracture of the humerus

Head and neck

Fractures of those portions known as the **surgical neck** and the **tuberosities** of the humerus are common, particularly in elderly people (Fig. 20.11).

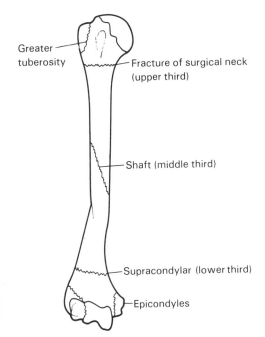

Greater tuberosity

Fracture of surgical neck (upper third)

Shaft (middle third)

Supracondylar (lower third)

Epicondyles

Fig. 20.11 Common fractures of the humerus.

History. The force is usually indirect and follows a fall onto the outstretched arm.

Symptoms and signs. The patient complains of pain and inability to move the arm and, as in all fractures of the upper limb, finds it necessary to support the weight of the limb with the other arm. This fracture is often associated with a dislocation of the shoulder, which is a very serious injury, when the patient may be in shock. The diagnosis is based on the pain, loss of power and tenderness. When this fracture is impacted, other physical signs are not usually seen.

Treatment. A broad bandage is applied first, to hold the arm to the side of the body. The weight of the arm can then be taken by a triangular sling. Frequently a collar-and-cuff bandage is all that is required (Fig. 20.12).

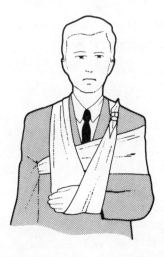

Fig. 20.12 Fracture of upper third of humerus: alternative treatment.

Middle third of the humerus

History. Injury follows a fall or direct blow to the arm.

Symptoms and signs. This fracture usually shows the classical signs of a fracture. There is pain, swelling and deformity. The arm is frequently in an abnormal position and crepitus is often complained of by the patient.

Treatment. A collar-and-cuff bandage will support the wrist at the neck. The arm is stabilized against the trunk by using a broad bandage. The weight of the arm in this case is applying a little traction to the fracture, which is a useful thing.

Supracondylar fracture

History. This fracture, near the elbow, occurs commonly in children and is often seen following a fall from a swing.

Symptoms and signs. There is usually pain, swelling, bruising, deformity and inability to use the elbow.

Treatment. It is a serious fracture with the possibility of injury to the blood vessels in the elbow. The arm should be well padded and supported in a triangular sling. If the arm is extended when the patient is seen and the pulse is satisfactory, then the arm should be supported by a well-padded splint in this position. Finger extension should be tested frequently – if this is painful or limited the splintage should be checked and the patient moved to hospital urgently.

Ulna: fractured olecranon

History. This is usually fractured by a direct injury to the upper ulna, i.e. in a fall on the point of the elbow.

Symptoms and signs. The patient complains of pain and inability to extend the arm, and is usually supporting the weight of the forearm. Frequently a gap can be felt between the two fragments in the early stage of this fracture.

Treatment. A well-padded splint is used to immobilize the fracture in the position which the casualty finds most comfortable.

Radius: fracture of the neck of the radius

History. This is common and again can follow a fall onto the outstretched arm.

Symptoms and signs. The patient complains of pain with inability to rotate the arm. There is usually some interference with full flexion and extension.

Treatment. A triangular sling should be applied.

Fracture of the radius and ulna

History. These two bones are frequently fractured together in the forearm, either by a direct or indirect blow (Fig. 20.13). In children they are commonly seen as greenstick fractures.

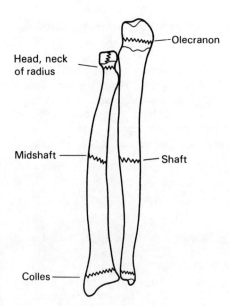

Head, neck
of radius

Olecranon

Midshaft

Shaft

Colles

Fig. 20.13 Fractures of radius and ulna.

Symptoms and signs. Pain, swelling, deformity, inability to use the arm are present, and the patient is normally supporting the injured limb.

Treatment. Application of a well-padded splint with a triangular sling to support the limb is required. When a splint is not available, the arm should be put in a sling and held against the body by a broad bandage to avoid excess movement during the journey to hospital.

Fracture of the shaft of the ulna

This fracture is occasionally seen, usually following a direct blow. The treatment is as for both forearm bones.

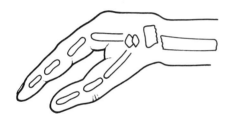

Fig. 20.14 Colles' fracture (dinner fork deformity).

Colles' fracture

History. This is one of the commonest fractures and usually follows a fall on the outstretched hand (Fig. 20.14).

Symptoms and signs. There is a typical 'dinnerfork' deformity at the lower wrist, with pain, swelling and tenderness over the fracture site and inability to use the hand.

Treatment. The fracture is usually impacted and is therefore stable. A triangular sling and a padded splint should be applied if the patient has to travel a long distance to hospital.

Scaphoid fracture

History. This bone in the wrist is commonly fractured following a fall.

Symptoms and signs. These consist of pain and swelling, with tenderness in the 'anatomical snuff-box' which is on the side of the wrist at the base of the thumb.

Treatment. This fracture is often missed during the early stages, as the signs are similar to sprains of the wrist. Repeated x-ray investigation may be required. First aid should be directed to making the patient comfortable with a sling.

Fractures of the metacarpals

History. Such fractures frequently follow injury in a fall, or fighting: in industrial accidents they are associated with compound injuries (Fig. 20.15).

Symptoms and signs. The simple fractures show pain, swelling, bruising and tenderness over the line of the metacarpal with interference of hand

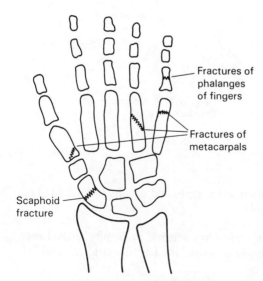

Fractures of
phalanges
of fingers

Fractures of
metacarpals

Scaphoid
fracture

Fig. 20.15 Fractures of the wrist and hand.

function. When looking at the back of the hand, there will be shortening of the knuckle.

Treatment. For first aid, a sling is usually all that is required: however, if it is an open injury, a dressing will be needed as well.

Fractures of the phalanges

These are often difficult to differentiate from dislocation. The easiest first aid technique is to strap the injured finger to the adjacent one.

FRACTURES OF THE LOWER LIMB

Fractures of the lower limb are often associated with more severe injury and with more blood in the fracture haematoma. In the case of the pelvis internal injury often occurs, and the signs of shock should be carefully looked for. First aid treatment of the fractures of the leg is directed towards using the other limb as a splint. Moderate angulation or deformity can often be corrected by gentle traction: pads are then applied between the ankles and the knees. The feet and ankles are tied together with a figure-of-eight bandage, both knees tied together with a broad bandage, and finally another broad bandage above and one below the fracture.

Fracture of the pelvis

History. This is a strong bone whose structure is designed to resist the body weight and the force of the lower limb (Fig. 20.16). Therefore it takes quite a lot of force to fracture it and, because of the degree of trauma required, the risk of damage to internal organs is considerable.

Symptoms and signs. Shock should be carefully looked for, and regular observations should be made of the patient's general condition and pulse. The patient should be lying down; gentle examination will show bruising, swelling and localized tenderness. Pressure on the bones by placing the hands on either side of the pelvis and gently pressing together will frequently cause pain, as does movement of the leg. The abdomen will often be bruised and can show tenderness. The muscles will contract and become hard on gentle pressure – this is called 'guarding' and is a sign of severe injury.

Complications. One of the most common complications is rupture of the bladder or urethra, the tube along which the urine passes. There is pain, bruising and swelling in the perineum, and if the patient passes water this could leak through the urethra into the surrounding tissue. If the patient wants to pass water it is advisable to ask him to restrain until he is seen in hospital. Occasionally damage to the rectum will occur; in such cases blood passes out of the anus.

Damage to the many blood vessels in the pelvis will cause internal haemorrhage and produce the signs of shock – pallor, restlessness, falling blood pressure and rising pulse rate.

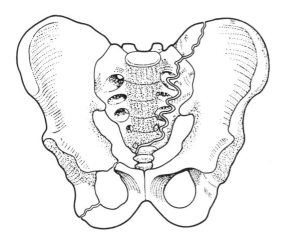

Fig. 20.16 Fractured pelvis. Note fracture on left side extending through sacrum; also two fractures on right side.

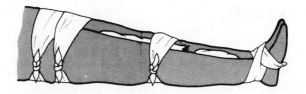

Fig. 20.17 Treatment of fractured pelvis.

Treatment. Speedy evacuation to hospital is required. The legs should be bound together and the patient moved on a stretcher if possible (Fig. 20.17). The patient must not be given anything by mouth.

Fractures of the femur

Upper end of the femur

History. The femur is frequently fractured at the neck or through the trochanters (Fig. 20.18). Fractures of the neck are more common in the

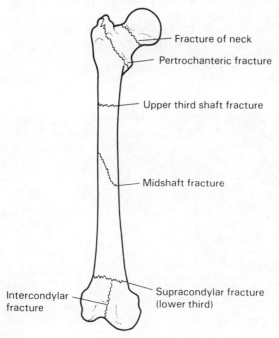

Fracture of neck

Pertrochanteric fracture

Upper third shaft fracture

Midshaft fracture

Intercondylar fracture

Supracondylar fracture (lower third)

Fig. 20.18 Fractures of the femur.

elderly because of bone rarefaction. Trochanteric fractures may occur at any age.

Symptoms and signs. The fracture through the base of the neck may be an impacted fracture with minimal signs other than pain, limp and shortening of the leg. There may be some delay in diagnosis because of the few signs. Femoral neck fractures, or trochanteric fractures, usually have more pain; there is shortening of the leg and the foot is frequently rotated outwards.

Treatment. The patient can be made comfortable by laying him down with his knees padded and a broad bandage applied around them. The lateral rotation should be gently corrected. A figure-of-eight bandage applied to the ankles will be sufficient to control the fracture. Many patients find it more comfortable to have the hip flexed over a pillow or a coat.

Shaft of the femur

History This is a much more serious injury; the bone is thicker, there is more muscle damage and the force required is greater. Considerable direct or indirect trauma will be described by patient or onlookers.

Symptoms and signs are therefore much more obvious. There will be severe pain, swelling, shortening of the limb and external rotation of the foot. Deformity may be obvious with the combination of shortening and angulation. Comminuted fractures will produce more damage; there will be more bleeding and therefore the incidence of shock will be greater.

Condylar fractures

T-shaped fractures frequently occur and split the condyles. This naturally involves the knee joint, and there is a painful swelling of the knee as well as the other signs of fracture. The knee has a tense, swollen collection of blood in the joint which is very painful.

Treatment. Fractures of the shaft of the femur will be associated with more severe loss of blood. The patient may be in shock, so urgent attention must be directed towards this. In road traffic accidents the presence of a wound, making this an open fracture, will require a dressing to be applied first. Gentle traction on the feet with medial rotation (towards the midline) will enable the ankles to be bound together by a figure-of-eight bandage (Figs. 20.19 and 20.20). Further broad bandages should be applied around the knee, above and below the fracture and around the middle of the legs. Long padded splints, when available, should be applied (see Fig. 20.32). It is applied to the outer side of the broken limb, extending from the armpit to the

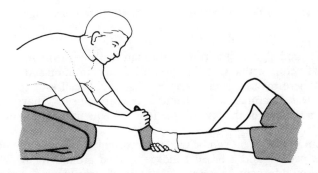

Fig. 20.19 Fractured femur: treatment (first stage). Supporting the foot and applying extension. Note: the sound leg has been bent to facilitate demonstration. An assistant should steady the patient.

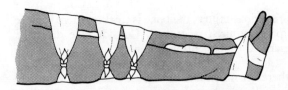

Fig. 20.20 Treatment of fractured femur (completed).

foot. Care must be taken that the bandages are firm and the fracture is properly splinted and cannot move in transit. The patient must be carefully lifted onto the stretcher using at least three people.

Thomas's splint. Efficient traction controls the ends of the fractured femur. Lives will be saved by the application of Thomas's type splint, particularly if the injury is open or associated with a bomb or missile injury, and if the patient has to travel a long distance. When first introduced, in World War I, the Thomas's splint reduced mortality from open femoral fractures from 80% to 20%. Condylar fractures may also be treated with Thomas's splint (Fig. 20.21).

Fracture of the patella

History. Fracture of the patella (Fig. 20.22) is common and usually follows a direct blow. Occasionally it will occur from strong muscle action, particularly if the bone has been affected by the long term use of steroid drugs. The fracture may be stellate (star shaped) or transverse.

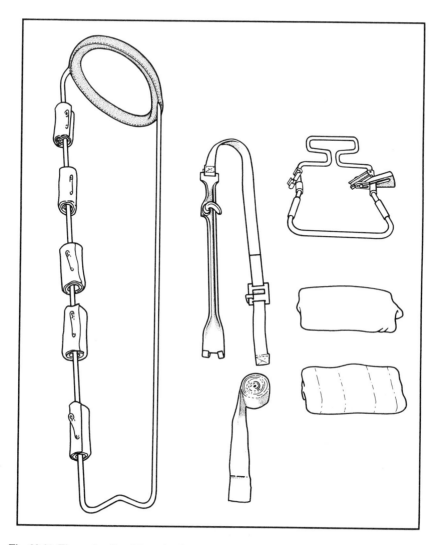

Fig. 20.21 Thomas's splint. Note: the ring in this pattern is well padded and specially shaped to fit the thigh. Usually, in first aid, the ring is a pure oval so that the splint can be used for either limb. With thanks to Brigadier RG Robinson.

Symptoms and signs. The stellate fracture is often associated with a marked effusion (swelling due to fluid) but there is no separation of the fragments. The knee is painful and swollen, with tenderness over the patella. The transverse fracture will have separation of the fragments and the patient will

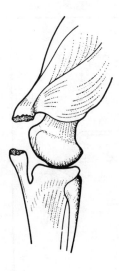

Fig. 20.22 Fracture of patella. Note displacement of fragments.

be unable to straighten the leg. A painful, tense swelling of the knee joint will occur. With car accidents look at the driver's hip – often there is an associated dislocation which can be missed.

Treatment. Gently straighten the leg and fasten this to the other leg using broad bandages above and below the joint. The ankles should be tied with the figure-of-eight bandage. Care must be taken when applying bandages near the knee, as the effusion will become greater and constriction must be avoided. This is the reason for a lot of padding and careful observation of the circulation below the fracture.

Fractures of the tibia

History. Fractures of the upper plateau of the tibia are associated with damage to the ligaments and with blood in the knee joint. The common car-bumper fracture produces a depressed fracture of the upper table of the tibia on the lateral side with damage to the medial and cruciate ligaments of the knee joint.

Symptoms and signs. Severe pain, inability to stand, tense swollen knee joint. The first aid **treatment** is similar to the condylar and patellar fractures.

Fractures of shaft of tibia

History. The tibia is easily felt under the skin of the shin, so fractures are frequently associated with damage to the overlying skin. Care must be taken when dealing with this fracture to avoid making it into an open fracture. The fractures are *transverse* from direct injury, *spiral* from indirect, or *oblique* from a combination of these (Fig. 20.23). Comminution is not uncommon in road traffic accidents, particularly those involving motor cyclists.

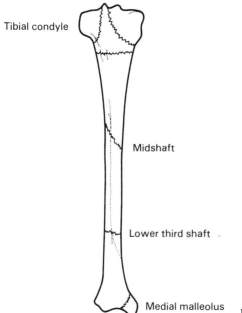

Tibial condyle

Midshaft

Lower third shaft

Medial malleolus

Fig. 20.23 Fractures of tibia.

Symptoms and signs. The leg is painful with bruising, swelling and tenderness. Deformity with angulation and rotation of the foot may be seen. Commonly, an open wound with protruding bone will be seen. Signs of shock are often present.

Treatment. The limb should be gently straightened and rotated, so that the ankles can be bound together with a figure-of-eight bandage. Dressing should be applied to the wounds, and broad bandages applied above and below the fracture, after placing padding between the legs. The knees should be bound

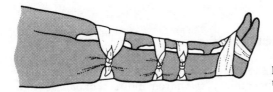

Fig. 20.24 Treatment of fractured leg.

together (Fig. 20.24). This fracture, and Pott's fracture described below, is
best treated with the inflatable splint (see below) which is now readily
available at many sports centres, outdoor sporting activities and first aid
centres, and is carried by most ambulances (see Fig. 20.29).

Ankle fractures

History. Fractures of the lateral and medial malleoli (Pott's Fractures) are
extremely common and are difficult to differentiate from a severe sprain of
the ankle (Fig. 20.25).

Symptoms and signs. There is pain, inability to walk, swelling and bruising,
and in a severe injury the foot may be displaced. Simple first degree fractures
of the lateral malleolus may only be detected by x-ray examination, as the
patient is able to walk on them. Careful examination should show tenderness
on the bone over the fracture site. This can be felt about 4 cm above the tip of
the lateral malleolus and 2 cm above the tip of the medial malleolus. In the
case of the sprain the tenderness is below the tip of the bone on either side.

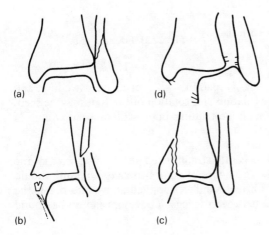

Fig. 20.25 Varieties of Pott's
fractures of the ankle: (a) fracture of lateral malleolus; (b) fracture of lateral and medial malleoli; (c) fracture of medial malleolus; (d) subluxation of joint
with tearing of ligaments (plus
fracture of neck of fibula).

Treatment. An inflatable splint or figure-of-eight binding of the two ankles and feet is required.

Fractures of the foot (Fig. 20.26)

Fractures of the heel

History. Fractures of the heel bone, the os calcis, are common after falling from a height.

Symptoms and signs. The heel is swollen and painful, and the patient is unable to put pressure on his heel and walks with difficulty.

Fractures of the talus

History. These occur with motor cycle accidents or severe twisting injury, sometimes with dislocation.

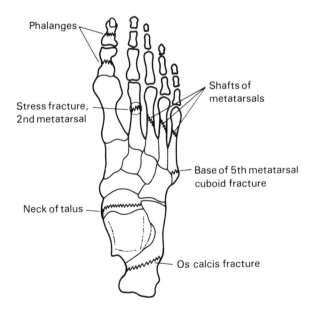

Phalanges

Shafts of
metatarsals

Stress fracture,
2nd metatarsal

Base of 5th metatarsal
cuboid fracture

Neck of talus

Os calcis fracture

Fig. 20.26 Fractures of bones of the foot.

Symptoms and signs. There is gross bruising and swelling of the middle of the foot.

Fractures of the metatarsals

History. These occur following direct or indirect injury. Fractures of the fifth metatarsal on the outside of the foot occur frequently when the foot is twisted.

Symptoms and signs. There is localized bruising, swelling and tenderness over the affected bone. Stress fractures of metatarsals are common in joggers, marchers and marathon runners.

With damage to the mid-tarsal joint, observation of the circulation in the toenails should be made, and if this is poor, urgent evacuation to a hospital is required.

Fractures of the phalanges

History. These occur after a direct blow or following a kicking action or stubbing the toes.

Symptoms and signs. There is bruising, swelling and tenderness.

Treatment

With fractures of the foot the boot should be left on, and the two feet bound together. Open injuries will require a dressing; in such cases a supporting bandage is usually adequate. The common toe fractures can be treated easily by strapping the toes together.

TREATMENT OF FRACTURES BY SPLINTS

General principles

A splint may be defined as any appliance which is capable of restricting the movement of an injured part.

Splints are extensively employed in first aid. Their use calls for practice on the part of the first aider; unless they are efficiently applied the patient may suffer shock due to careless handling of the injury. Moreover, the time taken in their application may delay his removal to shelter. For these reasons, modern teaching is that simple methods should be used whenever possible.

Nevertheless, there are still occasions when splints are essential, so every advanced first aider should be familiar with the methods which are described in this chapter.

Uses

The main object of splinting as a first aid procedure is to prevent a fracture becoming compound or complicated during transport; splints also provide complete rest to an injured part, and so relieve pain and encourage healing.

Indications for use of splints

It is difficult to lay down hard and fast rules as to when splints should be employed instead of body-splinting, and in every case the first aider must use his discretion depending on the circumstances which prevail at the accident. In general, the following are indications for the use of splints:
1. When the injured limb cannot satisfactorily be supported against a sound part of the body.
2. When there is likely to be considerable delay before medical services become available.
3. When the distance to hospital is long.
4. When the patient has to be carried over uneven ground.

Types available

Wooden. Straight pieces of wood of varying lengths and widths are often used in first aid.

Metal. Splints made of tin and aluminium are usually moulded as a gutter, to fit the natural curvatures of a limb, and padded with felt. They are ready for immediate use.

Wire. Cramer's wire splinting is also popular (Fig. 20.27). It can be quickly cut to the required length and easily bent to support a limb in any desired position. It is made of a framework of metal, strengthened by struts and curved from side to side to fit the limbs.

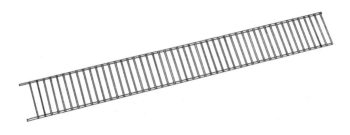

Fig. 20.27 Cramer's wire splinting. Courtesy of FW Equipment Co Ltd.

Plaster. Plaster of Paris (POP) is often used by surgeons in the treatment of fractures. Special splints can quickly be made to suit individual cases. Roller bandages of 4 or 6 inch widths are used for this purpose, made from a material with a coarse mesh which is filled with powdered plaster of Paris. They are soaked in water for a few seconds before use.

To make a plaster of Paris splint, a bandage is unrolled onto a smooth surface and folded eight times upon itself to form a slab of desired length. After immersing in water it is gently squeezed, moulded upon the affected part and secured in position by a roller bandage (used wet). When the plaster sets, it becomes hard and forms an excellent splint. The POP slab can be applied as a U-slab, thus giving support on both sides of the limb.

Note. Plaster of Paris slabs with a crepe paper bandage can be obtained as an emergency splint pack in a polythene bag (Fig. 20.28).

Inflatable splints. The inflatable splint is widely used in first aid and is an essential piece of equipment in the accident ambulance. It is quick and easy to apply and extremely comfortable for the patient (Fig. 20.29).

Inflatable splints are easy to apply but they are frequently misused. Inflation should be done by mouth. If a pump is used there is a real danger of over-inflation and constriction. When used for a fracture of the lower limb it

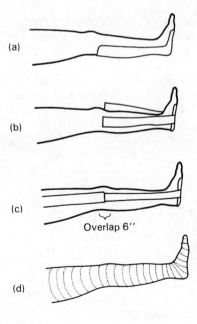

(a)

(b)

(c)

Overlap 6''

(d)

Fig. 20.28 Application of POP emergency slabs for fractures of tibia or ankle: (a) apply back slab; (b) apply U-slab; (c) extend for fractures of tibia; (d) damp paper crepe bandage.

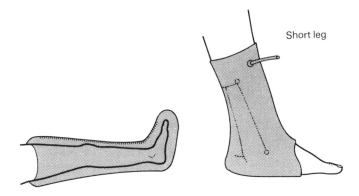

Short leg

Fig. 20.29 The inflatable splint. Courtesy of FW Equipment Co Ltd.

should never be applied over a boot or sock, as it is essential to keep the circulation of the foot under constant observation. It is particularly important to take care not to occlude the circulation in elderly patients.

Frequently the splint may partially deflate, at which point it ceases to act as a splint. This is invariably due to an inadequately secured valve, so attention should be paid to the correct technique.

The splint should not be used for air evacuation at altitudes above 1000 metres, as expansion of the contained air may cause serious damage to the limb.

Vacuum splints. These are more suitable for evacuation by air.

Box splint. Splints of PVC-covered wood, ready-padded, constructed on the box principle and rapidly fastened with velcro straps, are an efficient modern method of splinting (Fig. 20.30).

Body splinting. This is an effective method in many fractures. The techniques using broad bandages have been discussed above. Broad straps of

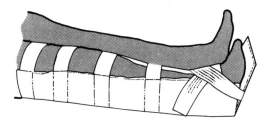

Fig. 20.30 Box splint. Courtesy of Loxley Medical.

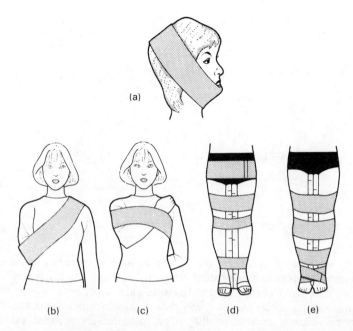

Fig. 20.31 Body splinting using Frac straps: (a) treatment for fractured jaw; (b) treatment for fractured humerus; (c) treatment for fractured collar bone; (d) treatment for hip or femur injury; (e) treatment for tibia and fibula with two short straps joined for figure-of-eight bandage. Courtesy of FW Equipment Co Ltd.

PVC-coated nylon (which maintain tension by means of elasticated panels) have the advantage of being easily applied (Fig. 20.31). They can be used in conjunction with wooden splints or PVC-padded splints (Fig. 20.32).

Application of splints

There are a number of important points to remember in the use and application of splints.

Choice. The splints chosen should be sufficiently strong and of a suitable length and width. The splint should be long enough to keep the joints immediately above and below the fracture at rest.

Padding. The splint should be covered with cotton wool or polythene foam. Padding is necessary to prevent discomfort or damage to the skin by pressure from the hard splint. Splints can be applied over the clothing, which will then act as a temporary padding.

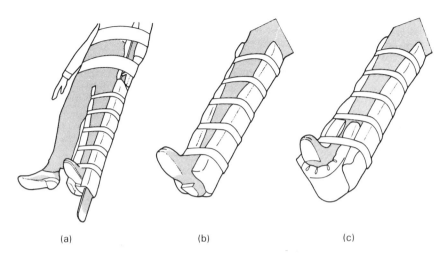

(a)   (b)   (c)

Fig. 20.32 PVC padded splints: (a) long leg splint (using Frac-straps) and wooden splint; (b) short leg splint; (c) foot splint. Courtesy of FW Equipment Co Ltd.

Moulding. When a choice of splints is possible, choose one which is most suitably moulded to fit the natural curvature of the limb.

Fixation. Splints must be fixed to the injured limb by bandages placed above and below the fracture, according to the following rules:
1. A bandage should never be allowed to encircle the limb at the actual site of the fracture, owing to the risk of causing complications; for this reason it is desirable to apply the bandages well above and below the seat of injury.
2. The bandage above the fracture is always tied before the one below.
3. Additional bandages may be employed to ensure fixation; when the lower limb is broken it is usual, after splinting, to tie the injured limb to its fellow of the opposite side, which acts as an extra safeguard while the patient is being removed to hospital.
4. Narrow bandages are generally used to fix splints to a limb, but if a splint is to be secured to the trunk, as in the treatment of a fractured femur, broad bandages should be employed.

Observation. After the application of splints and bandages, the first aider must satisfy himself that the circulation of the limb is still active. The pulse should be felt whenever possible, and careful watch should be kept on the fingernails and toenails, which will be found to change their colour to a blue or whitish hue if the bandages have been applied too tightly.

Rings, bracelets and watches should be removed from an injured arm or hand.

Improvisation of splints

In an emergency when regular splints are unobtainable, they must be improvised from any suitable articles which are to hand. Thus, walking sticks, umbrellas, billiard cues, broomsticks or even rolls of cardboard can be used as temporary splints. Bandages to secure them into position can similarly be improvised from ties, scarves, belts or even stockings; the improvisation of suitable appliances is a challenge to the imagination of the first aider.

Fractures of the upper extremity

Fractures of the humerus

The only fracture of the humerus likely to require splints is one in which the shaft of the bone has been broken. Occasionally, however, an angular splint is used for fractures near the elbow.

Shaft of the humerus

Method:
1. Place the arm on the affected side in a small arm sling (Fig. 20.33).
2. Place in position two narrow bandages as follows:
   (a) carefully guide the first bandage through the armpit and allow its upper end to hang over the shoulder.

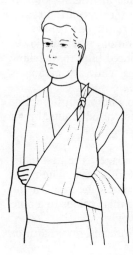

Fig. 20.33 Fracture of middle third of humerus: before applying splints.

(b) place the second bandage through the bend of the elbow.

3. Obtain three splints of suitable length and apply them to the arm, so that they extend from the shoulder to the elbow along the front, outside and back of the limb in its present position. Arrange for the splints to be supported in this position.

4. Collect the ends of the upper bandage and carry them twice round the arm and the splints, above the level of the fracture; tie them on the outer splint.

5. Similarly collect the ends of the lower bandage and carry them twice round the arm and splints, below the level of the fracture, and tie them on the outer splint so that the second knot is in line with the first. Tuck the ends neatly away (Fig. 20.34).

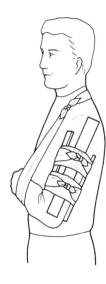

Fig. 20.34 Fracture of middle third of humerus: treatment completed. Note: the splint along the front of the arm has been slightly turned outwards in order to show it up.

Notes.

1. The faces of the splints should be at right angles to each other.

2. Care must be taken that the bandages which secure the splint to the arm are well above and below the level of the fracture.

Lower third of the humerus

Angular splint method. This consists of the application of a special splint, known as a right-angled splint, which ensures that the forearm is kept at right angles to the arm. An angular splint, however, is not often obtainable when

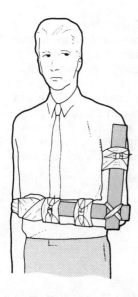

Fig. 20.35 Angular splint applied before putting arm in sling.

required, and must therefore be improvised by taking two splints of suitable length and knotting them together to form a right angle (Fig. 20.35). An improvised splint has the advantage that it can easily be adjusted to suit the size of the arm. Cramer wire or POP slabs are particularly suitable (Fig. 20.36).

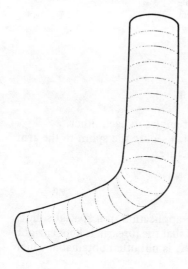

Fig. 20.36 Cramer wire splint for fractures near the elbow joint.

1. Gently bend up the patient's forearm (keeping the thumb uppermost) until it is nearly at right angles to the arm. Support the forearm in this position. Feel the pulse to make certain that the circulation is not impeded. If it is, lower the forearm to less than a right angle.

2. Apply the angular splint to whichever side of the elbow shows less swelling.

3. Secure the splint in position by three bandages as follows:
    (a) one taken twice round the middle of the arm,
    (b) one taken twice round the middle of the forearm, and
    (c) a figure-of-eight bandage around the wrist and hand.

4. Place the arm on the affected side in a large arm sling.

5. Occasionally supracondylar fractures need to be splinted in extension. Be guided by the position of the limb, degree of swelling and the radial pulse. The splintage is then similar to that for fractured olecranon below.

Fractured olecranon

Treatment.
1. Apply a splint along the front of the limb, extending from the upper third of the arm to the palm of the hand, to prevent bending of the elbow (Fig. 20.37).

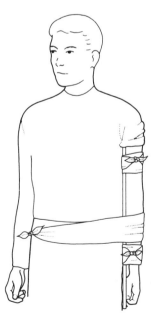

Fig. 20.37 Treatment of fractured olecranon.

2. Secure the splint in position by two bandages, as follows:
   (a) the first taken twice round the middle of the arm and tied on the side of the limb.
   (b) the second taken twice round the forearm and tied on the side of the forearm.
3. Secure the limb to the side of the body by a broad bandage passed round the forearm and the trunk, and then tied on the sound side.

Fracture of the forearm

Treatment.
1. Gently bend up the patient's forearm until it is at right angles to the arm, keeping the thumb uppermost (Figs. 20.38 and 20.39). Support the limb in this position.
2. Apply padded splints to the front and back of the forearm extending from the elbow to the fingers.

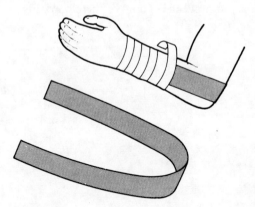

Fig. 20.38 Plaster of Paris U-slab.

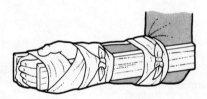

Fig. 20.39 Fractured forearm: treatment before application of sling.

3. Secure the splints in position by two bandages as follows:
    (a) one above the level of the fracture, taken twice round the forearm and tied on the outer splint, and
    (b) one around the wrist and hand as a figure-of-eight.
4. Apply a large arm sling.

Note. The splint along the palm side of the forearm should extend to the level of the fingertips, but the one along the back of the forearm should stop short just beyond the last joint of the fingers, so that the nails remain visible and any change in their colour which would suggest impeded circulation, can be noted.

Fracture of the hand

Treatment.
1. Place sterile pad over wound (Fig. 20.40).

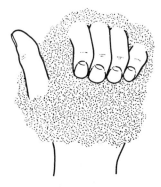

Fig. 20.40 Treatment of fracture of the hand: stage one.

2. Fluffed-up gauze is placed in the palm and between the thumb and index finger.
3. If wool bandage is available, a layer of wool is added.
4. Crepe bandage is applied over the fingers, leaving a hole for the thumb to protrude. The object is to keep the fingers straight. Then bandage the palm and wrist (Fig. 20.41).
5. A well-padded splint or POP slab can be applied on the palm aspect up to the level of the fingers.

Note. If one phalanx only is broken, a small, well-padded splint may be temporarily placed along the palm side of the finger, and secured in position by strips of adhesive plaster above and below the fracture.

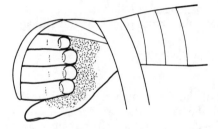

Fig. 20.41 Treatment of fracture of the hand: stage two.

Fractures of the lower limb

Fracture of the femur

Treatment.
Side splint method.
1. Support the foot on the injured side by placing one hand over the instep and the second under the ankle. Gentle traction is applied and the leg is brought into line.
2. Apply a well-padded splint between the limbs extending from the groin to the feet.
3. Tie both feet and ankles together by a figure-of-eight bandage to include this splint. This begins behind the ankles and the ends are brought upwards and crossed over insteps; they are then carried under the soles of the feet and tied in this situation, using a surgeon's knot for the purpose.
4. Pass a series of seven folded bandages under the patient's body so that they come to lie in certain definite places. All the bandages are placed under the patient without moving his body. Each bandage is folded over a splint, which is then passed from the injured side under the patient's body, and one end of the bandage pulled through on the sound side. The natural hollows of the body are used wherever possible. Thus, two bandages can be passed under the hollow of the small of the back; another just below the buttocks; other natural hollows include the backs of the knees and the ankles. After passing the bandages under the body in these places, they should be worked upwards or downwards until they come to lie in the appropriate positions as shown in Fig. 20.42, that is:

Number 2   Under the chest, just below the level of the armpits.
Number 3   Under the hips.
Number 4   Under both ankles.
Number 5   Under both thighs, above the level of the fracture.
Number 6   Under both thighs, below the level of the fracture.
Number 7   Under the legs.

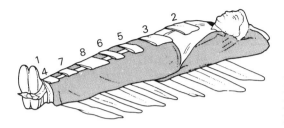

Fig. 20.42 Fractured femur: treatment. All the bandages have now been passed under the patient.

Number 8   Under the knees.

All these bandages should be narrow, except those placed under the chest, hips and knees, which should be of the broad variety.

5. Place a second, long splint along the injured side of the patient, extending from the armpit to the foot. The splint may be padded where it is liable to dig into the armpit, and also at the side of the knee.

6. Secure the splint in position by tying the bandages in the same order as that in which they were passed. All the bandages should be tied on the centre of the splint except the one under the ankles; this must be applied as a figure-of-eight and tied under the soles of the feet, thus covering the first bandage which was used to secure the feet and ankles together (Fig. 20.43).

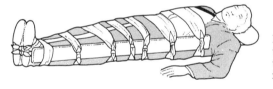

Fig. 20.43 Fractured femur: treatment completed. Note the two knots under the soles of the feet.

Notes.

1. As far as possible the bandages should be kept free from wrinkles and creases. This can be accomplished quite easily by keeping a steady tension on each bandage as it is brought round the body and tied on the splint.

2. All knots, with the exception of that of the bandage round the feet and ankles, are tied on the centre of the outer splint. The ends should be neatly tucked away.

Thomas's splint

Thomas's splint is still the most effective method of splinting the fractured femur, or indeed any fracture of the lower limb except the patella. It should always be used for severe wounds. It can be applied without removing boots or shoes. Only if there is a wound need the trousers be split for applying a dressing.

The advantage of Thomas's splint is that the limb is fixed so that the bony fragments of the fracture are not jolted against one another during a rough or prolonged journey. It does, however, take time to apply as there are many bits and pieces to collect and additional helpers are necessary (see Fig. 20.21).

The principle is that the padded ring of the splint is wedged firmly in the groin pressing on the ischial tuberosity of the pelvis. From this purchase the leg is extended between the side arms of the splint and secured to the notch in the narrower end. Support of the limb is achieved by lengths of wide bandages secured transversely by safety pins between the sides of the splint.

Application.
1. Three people are required to apply the splint:
   (a) the first aider, who applies the splint;
   (b) an assistant (Fig. 20.44), who maintains traction on the limb, holds the heel and toe of the patient's boot or shoe and exerts a steady pull (this pull must be continued without relaxation throughout the application);
   (c) a further assistant, who gives additional support by placing his hands under the limb on either side of the fracture.
2. To make a clove hitch:
   (a) take about 3 m of broad flannel bandage;
   (b) fold at one-third of its length and place across the ankle (Fig. 20.45) with the loop on the inner side;
   (c) the two free ends, one short, one long, are taken through the loop;
   (d) the longer end is passed beneath the instep and under both the loops on the outer side;

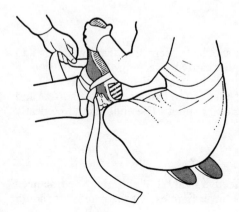

Fig. 20.44 Clove hitch being applied; assistant maintains traction.

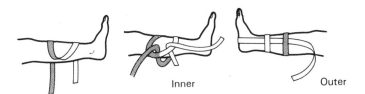

Inner   Outer

Fig. 20.45 Clove hitch.

    (e) the knot is made reasonably secure.

3. The splint is prepared by tying a broad bandage to its ring where this joins the outer bar, passing it over the inner bar, back to the outer bar and so on down the splint to form a supporting trough. Alternatively, five separate cross-supports can be made with separate lengths of wide bandage loosely secured by safety-pins along the length of the splint (Fig. 20.46).

4. The splint is now applied by passing the ring over the leg, the assistant releasing traction one hand at a time to allow this. The ring is pushed under the buttock as far as possible.

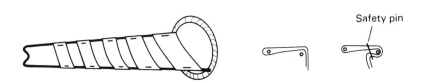

Safety pin

Fig. 20.46 Preparing cross supports.

5. The ends from the clove hitch are secured, the outer one passing over and under the bar and around the notch at the end of the splint, the inner one passing under and over the bar and round the notch where the two ends are drawn tight together and tied firmly in a half bow.

6. The limb is held down by a folded triangular bandage laid across the leg just below the knee. The ends are passed down between the leg and the splint, brought up outside it and tied off (Fig. 20.47).

7. Support for the end of the splint is provided by the rolled blanket which is placed across the stretcher beneath it. These may be further secured with a bandage.

8. Any wound should be finally dressed at this stage. Severe bleeding may need control from the start.

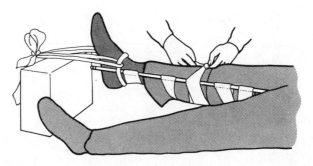

Fig. 20.47 Limb supported with clove hitch applied. Bandage which prevents leg from rising being tied.

9. Additional extension to the limb is obtained by means of the 'Spanish windlass'. This is simply a skewer or piece of wood passed down between the long ends of the clove hitch and twisted. The twist is maintained by leaving the skewer in place and allowing it to rest against the side of the splint.

Further support for the fractured femur may be obtained by placing two pieces of Cramer splinting along the front and back of the thighs, the back splint being the shorter. Both are held in place by bandages above and below the fracture.

10. Finally, if the ring is uncomfortable in the groin, additional padding (using cotton wool or other suitable material) may be introduced.

If available, a specially prepared stirrup may be used to secure the shoe to the sides of the splint to improve stability.

Instead of supporting the splint on a rolled blanket, an iron suspension bar made to fit the stretcher may be applied, from which the sling is strung by vertical and lateral bandages (Fig. 20.48).

Hare traction splint

Many modifications of Thomas's splint have been made to make its application easier. The same principle of traction with support of the limb is used in the Hare splint (Fig. 20.49). Modern materials are used to improve the speed of application and the splint's effectiveness. It is lightweight, compact and easy to store, requiring less space. The method of application is the same as the conventional Thomas's splint. A special traction cuff with velcro fastening fits around the ankle.

A positive traction device ensures the maintenance of the correct pressure without the risk of breaking the Spanish windlass. The thigh strap and leg

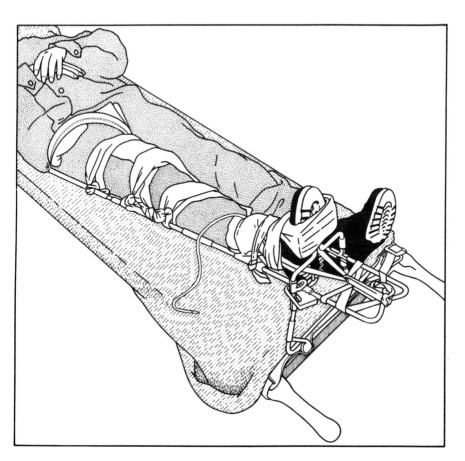

Fig. 20.48 Application of Thomas's splint: stages 1, 2 and completed. With thanks to Brigadier RG Robinson.

straps of protected nylon enable the splint to be fastened without disturbing the patient too much and reducing pain and shock. A neat heel stand supports the splint at the end of the operation.

Sager traction splint

The Sager traction splint has an advantage over the Thomas-type splint in that it can be very rapidly applied. It therefore overcomes the major resistance to traction splinting, i.e. the time involved to apply the splint.

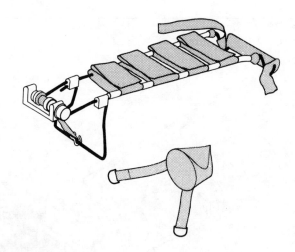

Fig. 20.49 Hare traction splint.

Fractures of the tibia and fibula

Treatment. The full-length inflatable splint is ideal for this injury.
    If this is not available treatment should be as follows:
1. Apply a well-padded splint between the limbs extending from the groin to the feet.
2. Bring the feet as nearly as possible into line without causing pain or using force.
3. Tie both feet and ankles together with a figure-of-eight bandage.
4. Apply a broad bandage round both thighs.
5. Bandage the knees together with a broad bandage.
6. Apply two bandages (narrow or broad, according to the size of the casualty) one above and one below the fracture (Fig. 20.50).

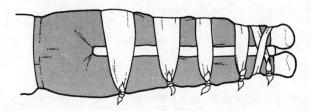

Fig. 20.50 Fractured leg: treatment completed without assistance.

Note. The bandages should be tied off over the uninjured limb when only one limb is affected, but over the side showing least injury when both limbs are fractured. In the case of a fracture near the ankle joint, the bandage nearest the joint may have to be omitted.

Fracture of the foot

Treatment (if a wound is present or suspected).
1. Remove the shoe and sock.
2. Treat the wound.
3. Apply a well-padded splint underneath the foot extending from the heel to the toe (Fig. 20.51).

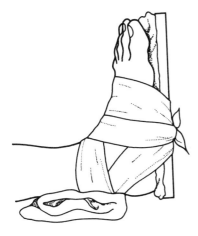

Fig. 20.51 Fractured foot.

4. Secure the splint in position by a narrow bandage. Place the centre of this bandage over the instep, carry the ends to the sole of the foot, and cross them over the splint. Then carry them to the back of the ankle and cross them again, bringing them to the front of the ankle. Cross them again, and finally pass them under the sole of the foot and tie on the splint.
5. Support the foot in an elevated position.

— 21

Injuries to the Joints and Muscles

INJURIES TO THE JOINTS

Joints, the moving articulations between the bones, are extremely susceptible to injury. The injury may damage the muscles at their attachment, the synovia, the capsule, the ligaments or the bones within the joint. Muscle injury equals strain or rupture; ligament injury equals sprain; bone injury equals fracture (Fig. 21.1).

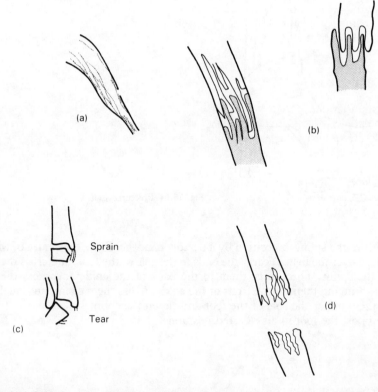

Fig. 21.1 Strains, sprains and tears: (a) muscle strain (similar tearing and partial separation of muscle fibres); (b) ligament sprain; (c) sprain and tear (joint will tilt with complete tear and is unstable); (d) ligament tear.

Some joints appear to be more vulnerable than others. These include the fingers, the elbow, shoulder, and ankle joints and the knee. An increase in the number of people playing sports has led to an increase in the number of injuries being sustained in and around joints: the first aider will be called upon more frequently to assess and treat these injuries. They will be seen early, which is an advantage, because at this time it is easier to feel the contour of the joint and to examine the ligaments before a large amount of swelling and bruising has occurred. Swelling within a joint occurring immediately after injury is usually due to haemorrhage following a complete tear of the capsule and synovia, whereas that following a sprain develops more slowly. In either case an increase is to be expected for 24 to 48 hours after the time of injury, and this must be taken into account during the treatment phase. The application of firm bandaging with cotton wool as padding will prevent oedema and swelling, but it is important that allowance is made for the extra swelling which will occur. The circulation of the fingers or toes must be watched carefully.

Joints which have been injured previously, or which are affected by osteoarthritis, are more liable to recurrent injury and effusion. This takes the form of synovitis, which may be troublesome particularly after minor injuries or overuse.

Sprains

A sprain around a joint will involve damage to fibres of the capsule which may extend into the ligaments or muscles. All degrees of injury, from a moderate sprain of the fibres (when the ligament or capsule is stretched) to a complete tear with rupture of the capsule and ligaments, may occur. When ligaments have been completely torn, the joint loses its stability. The joint is extremely vulnerable to recurrent dislocation if the ligaments are not properly repaired. The cause is usually indirect violence, in the form of wrenches or twists which force the joint too far in one particular direction.

History

The patient will describe the injury and can often explain how the joint was wrenched or twisted. He may even describe the ligaments giving way.

Symptoms and signs

Pain is initially localized to the site of the injury and is made worse by stretching the ligaments.

Loss of power is due to the pain but movement at the joint is still possible. Indeed the patient will often move the joint up and down to reassure himself that it is not dislocated.

Swelling and bruising: the time interval before their appearance is an indication of the severity of the damage to the ligaments and capsules around the joint, as described above.

Tenderness is felt initially over the soft tissues and not on the bone, except where the ligament's attachments have been torn (often with a small segment of bone attached).

Shock is not likely to occur but the pain will cause distress, or even fainting if severe.

Diagnosis

It is often difficult and in many cases an x-ray will be required to differentiate between sprain and fracture. If the tenderness is over the capsules and ligaments it is most likely a sprain, but if the tenderness is over the bone it is most likely a fracture. If in doubt treat as a fracture.

Treatment

Rest and elevation: the limb should be protected from further injury by rest, and should be elevated to decrease swelling. However, the muscles must be exercised to prevent wasting; this will also decrease the amount of swelling.

Application of a cold compress: a proprietary 'instant cold pack' or a bag containing crushed ice wrapped in a towel is placed on the swollen part of the limb.

A pressure bandage, that is a layer of cotton wool with a firm bandage over it, will restrict swelling. In the case of the larger joints, this may be supplemented by an extra layer each of cotton wool and bandage. The Robert Jones' bandage applied to the knee joint acts as a very firm splint, in addition to relieving pain and applying pressure. With this type of bandage it is important to elevate the limb and to watch the circulation of the toes. Crepe bandages are easy to apply, but again the circulation must be carefully observed. The modern cylindrical elastic bandage (e.g. Tubigrip®) is also very effective if applied double.

DISLOCATION

A dislocation is the displacement of the bony surfaces of the joint, and is associated with tearing of the capsule and ligaments. The cause is usually indirect violence, but occasionally (in the case of the jaw and kneecap) may be due to muscular overaction.

The classification of dislocations may be compared with that of fractures:
1. A **simple** dislocation is one in which the damage is restricted to the capsule and ligaments.
2. A **complicated** dislocation is one associated with damage to the nerves or adjacent blood vessels. This type of complication is particularly likely to happen at the elbow joint.
3. Dislocations are usually **closed**, but in severe cases with marked trauma, may also be associated with damage to the overlying skin. In such cases they are **open**. These are more likely to occur at the ankle joint, where the overlying skin is thin.
4. **Fracture dislocation** is a dislocation associated with a fracture. Fracture dislocations are common in the spine, elbow and ankle joints, and are a combination of tearing of the ligaments and displacement of the fractured bone ends; the fragments of bone are carried with the ligaments.

History

The history must be taken carefully, and is usually of a fall with indirect violence.

Symptoms and signs

Pain. This is severe in a dislocation, as joints are extremely sensitive. If there is pressure on surrounding nerves the pain may be felt down the limb. With pressure on blood vessels or prolonged pressure on nerves, the limb may become numb. Permanent damage may result.

Loss of power. Movement at the joint does not occur due to the displacement.

Swelling. The joint is immediately surrounded by an area of swelling and bruising due to the tear of the capsule and ligament.

Deformity. The affected joint will appear deformed when compared with its fellow on the opposite side.

Tenderness. There is tenderness around the joint associated with the torn capsule and ligaments. In the early phase before swelling has developed, the bone edges may be palpable; there will be irregularity of the bony points around the joint and often alteration in the length of the limb.

Diagnosis

It is often difficult to exclude fracture or fracture dislocation during the initial examination. In any case the important thing is to immobilize the limb and watch the circulation of the fingers or toes. The methods of splintage will be very much the same as those for a fracture. Early evacuation to a hospital is important, as x-rays and an anaesthetic will be required to reduce the displaced joint. The patient should not be given anything to drink.

Dislocations of specific joints

Only the more common dislocations are described below.

Shoulder

This is probably one of the commonest dislocations, and is seen frequently in sporting injuries (Fig. 21.2).

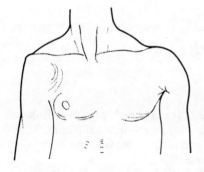

Fig. 21.2 Deformed shoulder due to dislocation. Note characteristic flattening of the right shoulder.

History. The patient has fallen forward and has put the arm out to protect himself. Pain is felt in the joint, associated with tearing sensations.

Symptoms and signs. Movements of the joint are prevented. On examination the normal contour of the shoulder has been lost. There is squaring of the joint and there is bruising and swelling on the front. Gentle palpation of the joint will reveal the prominent end of the clavicle and scapula with an empty glenoid socket where the head of the humerus should be. The head of the humerus is usually felt below the joint.

Treatment. The arm should be placed in a supporting sling and the patient taken to hospital for reduction of the dislocation. An anaesthetic will be required for relaxation of the muscle.

Elbow

History. This is usually of a fall, with the arm being placed awkwardly, followed by sudden pain and loss of movement of the elbow joint. Occasionally in children, swinging the child by the arms may dislocate the radial head of the joint.

Symptoms and signs. There is pain, swelling and inability to move the joint. The normal three-point plan of the two humeral epicondyles and the olecranon will be lost. This sign differentiates dislocation of the elbow from the common supracondylar fracture (Fig. 21.3), when the three bony points remain in the correct triangular position despite the other swelling and deformity (Fig. 21.4).

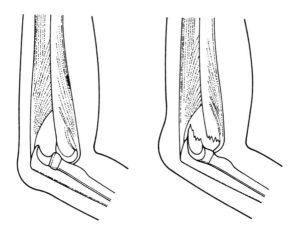

Fig. 21.3 Dislocation of elbow compared with fracture of lower end of humerus.

Finger

This joint is commonly dislocated in sports injuries, particularly at the proximal interphalangeal joint (Fig. 21.5). The finger is painful, stiff and extended, with the middle phalanx lying in front of the proximal phalanx and a palpable step between them. Early reduction is required, so the patient should be taken to a doctor as soon as possible. Splintage is not normally necessary but the arm may be more comfortable in a sling.

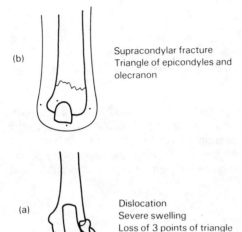

(b) Supracondylar fracture
Triangle of epicondyles and
olecranon

(a) Dislocation
Severe swelling
Loss of 3 points of triangle

Fig. 21.4 Dislocation/fracture
of elbow, indicating presence or
absence of the three points of the
elbow: (a) dislocation; (b) supracondylar fracture.

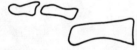

Fig. 21.5 Dislocation of finger.

Hip

Dislocations of the hip (Fig. 21.6) are serious injuries, as this is a very strong, well-protected joint.

History. They commonly appear in drivers of vehicles in road traffic accidents, and are often associated with fracture of the patella.

Symptoms and signs. The patient may be in shock, and will have severe pain and be unable to move the joint. There is shortening of the limb with inward (internal) rotation and adduction of the leg (the leg held against its fellow). The knee joint is often swollen, with tenderness over the kneecap.

Treatment. This is the same as for a fracture of the upper femur, as it is impossible without an x-ray to differentiate between them. Both limbs should

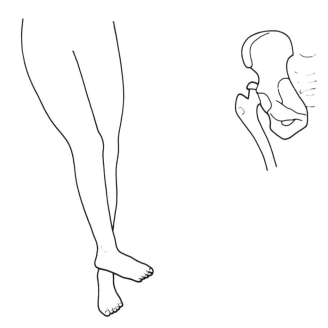

Fig. 21.6 Dislocation of hip.

be tied together with broad bandages (as for the fractured femur), and the patient transported on a stretcher to the nearest Accident and Emergency (A & E) Department. The limb should be supported on pillows for comfort.

Patella

History. Dislocations of the patella (Fig. 21.7) occur frequently, particularly as a sports injury in young women, when the kneecap goes to the outer side of the joint following a fall.

Symptoms and signs. The knee is bent and the kneecap can be felt on the outer side. Often a simple movement of extension of the joint will cause the kneecap to spring back into its normal position, then swelling will occur as an effusion of the joint develops.

Treatment. The legs should be bandaged together and the patient taken to the hospital for further investigation and treatment.

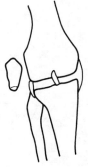

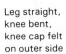

Leg straight,
knee bent,
knee cap felt
on outer side

Fig. 21.7 Dislocation of patella.

Knee

History. The knee is a strong joint, and dislocation (Fig. 21.8) occurs only after severe damage to the ligaments. Therefore it is associated with serious injury.

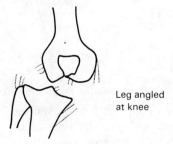

Leg angled
at knee

Fig. 21.8 Dislocation of knee.

Symptoms and signs. The patient is in severe pain and often in shock. Tearing of the ligaments will produce obvious deformity, swelling around the joint and loss of movement. Interference with the arteries and nerves may cause interference with the limb, producing coldness, absent pulse and loss of sensation.

Treatment. Fasten the limb (after it has been well padded) to the opposite leg. Urgent movement to a hospital is required for x-ray and reduction.

Ankle

History. Dislocations of the ankle are frequently associated with fractures of the malleoli as well as ligamentous tearing, and are thus technically fracture dislocations. The patient has had a severe injury, with rotational strain being applied to the joint after a fall.

Symptoms and signs. The ankle is painful and swollen and the foot is usually displaced backwards. This brings the lower end of the tibia into prominence, and the skin overlying this may become very white due to interference with blood supply.

Treatment. The limb should be well padded and a splint applied. Urgent transfer to a hospital is essential for x-ray and manipulation.

INJURIES TO MUSCLES

Injury to the muscle may be a strain or rupture of the muscle or its tendons. If excess force is applied to a muscle, like a severe twist, stretch or sudden exertion, muscle fibres may be torn. The damaged muscle starts to swell and, if the damage is severe, there may be bleeding into the main body of the muscle.

History

The patient will give a story of sudden onset of pain when performing a difficult movement, lifting or jumping, etc.

Symptoms and signs

Pain. This may be severe, and is aggravated by attempted movements.

Loss of power. This occurs when an attempt is made to use the muscle.

Tenderness. The muscle or its attachment is tender.

Swelling. This occurs fairly soon after the injury and may be followed by bruising, which may take some days to develop to its maximum.

Rupture. The rupture of the muscle fibres may commonly occur in the biceps or quadriceps. Initially a gap may be felt.

Treatment

Firstly, rest. The limb should be made comfortable and a sling applied so that the limb is elevated. A cold compress will relieve some of the pain and also reduce the amount of swelling. Once it is confirmed that there is no bony injury present, gentle graduated activity will further reduce the swelling and will restore muscle function. This will be assisted by the use of radiant heat, short wave diathermy, or ultra sound given by a physiotherapist. Contrast baths of cold and hot water will often help.

These injuries are particularly likely to occur as sports injuries, often at the beginning of a season, and can be avoided if progressive training is started well before matches are played, and if time is given for a warm-up before starting to play.

Ruptured tendons

Damage to a tendon occurs after sudden violence or a blow.
Some examples are:
1. The Achilles tendon is torn by a sudden effort, e.g. when playing squash, tennis or running. The patient complains of feeling a kick or sudden blow on the tendon and he loses the power of standing on his toes. Initially a gap can be felt and the tendon is painful and tender. This is a serious injury. The leg must be supported and medical advice sought at an early stage.
2. The extensor tendon on the back of the end joint of the finger is often injured in sport and the finger droops. This is called a 'mallet finger' and a special splint is required to keep it extended and straight.

Division of tendons

An incised or lacerated wound can involve the tendons running across a joint. It is important to assess movement of the joint and, in the case of the wrist, movement of the fingers and thumb. This is simple to do – the patient must be asked to flex and extend the fingers. This injury requires urgent surgical attention, so the wound must be dressed, a splint applied and the patient moved to hospital.

— 22

Spinal Injuries

The mobile spinal column is frequently injured: musculoligamentous and disc injury are some of the commonest causes of unfitness for work. Fracture or fracture dislocation of the vertebrae may irreparably damage the spinal cord. Characteristic features of most spinal injuries are rigidity, spasm and pain produced by damage to the muscles at the site of injury: if these are present, treat as for a fracture.

Structure

The bodies of the vertebrae are held together by strong intervertebral discs. The neural arch is attached to the back of the vertebral body; adjacent arches form a bony channel to protect the spinal cord (which passes through this channel within the dura mater). Each neural arch is connected, above and below, by the intervertebral joints and ligaments (see Fig. 22.1). Transverse

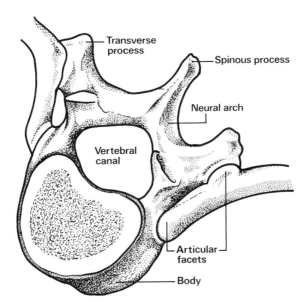

Fig. 22.1 Structure of typical vertebra.

191

processes on each side and a posterior spinous process are attached to the neural arch, are connected above and below by ligaments and have many muscular attachments. This posterior musculoligamentous complex, together with the strong vertebral disc attachment, is important for the stability of the spine.

Types of injury

Sprains of the ligaments occur as a result of forcible bending or sudden twists of the spine. Sudden severe pain is felt at the site of the injury, followed by tenderness, swelling and possibly bruising. Any movement makes the pain worse, particularly if the injured ligament is stretched. Strains of the attached muscles frequently occur at the same time as damage to the ligaments, so that it is difficult to differentiate between them. An example of this is whiplash injuries of the neck (Fig. 22.2) which commonly occur in car accidents, either if the car stops suddenly or is bumped from behind.

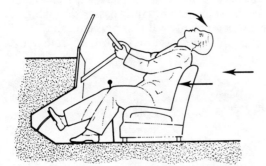

Fig. 22.2 Whiplash injury to neck.

Intervertebral disc. Prolapse or 'slipping' of the intervertebral disc may occur even after a trivial movement. The prolapsed disc is pressing on the spinal nerve as it passes between the vertebrae close to the disc. This causes back muscle spasm and severe pain, with inability to move. Disc prolapse is common in the neck and in the lumbar region.

1. Pressure on the nerve in the neck causes pain, often described as a funny feathery feeling down the arm, extending to one or other of the fingers.

2. In the lumbar region the pain will pass to the buttock and down the back of the leg, extending to the ankle in the common condition of sciatica.

Accurate diagnosis is often difficult in the early 'acute' phase after injury. Minor avulsion fractures, in which ligaments pull off their bony attachment, can only be detected by x-ray.

First aid treatment must be directed to making the patient comfortable. This will involve laying him down on a firm support and, in cases of injury to the neck, a cervical splint can be improvised from newspapers to rest the damaged soft tissues. A medical opinion should then be sought.

Fractures of the vertebrae. The important factor in these injuries is the stability of the vertebral column. If the vertebra itself is injured but the important posterior ligaments remain intact, then the fracture is stable and the spinal cord is protected. (This condition occurs with the common wedge fracture – see Fig. 22.3.) When these posterior ligaments have been torn in cases of vertebral fracture, then the injury is unstable. Movement of adjacent vertebrae is therefore possible and the spinal cord is at considerable risk. These fractures require great care when moving the patient, to avoid damage to the spinal cord.

Every suspected fracture of the vertebra should be treated as an unstable fracture to avoid risk to the spinal cord.

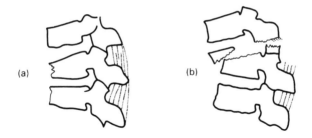

Fig. 22.3 Fractures of the vertebrae: (a) wedge fracture – stable; (b) fracture dislocation – unstable.

Causes of fracture

Strong muscular action can cause fractures of the spinous or transverse processes. Fractures of the spinous process of the seventh cervical vertebra (the 'shoveller's fracture') and the transverse processes of the lumbar vertebrae are the most common.

Direct violence, such as a severe blow on the head, or falling with the spine erect, may cause compression fractures of the vertebrae. If the disc is forced into the body of the vertebra, a burst fracture may occur. These fractures are stable, but the burst fracture may produce backward pressure onto the spinal cord.

Indirect violence, such as occurs in a heavy fall with a sudden bend, or diving into shallow water, or in a motor car collision when the head is jerked back forcibly over the top of the seat, causes the flexion and extension fractures. These commonly occur at the junction of the relatively immobile thoracic spine with the very mobile vertebrae in the lower part of the neck or the upper part of the lumbar spine. In the vast majority of these cases, the posterior ligament complex is intact so the spinal cord is protected. More severe violence may produce a shearing rotation injury, with tearing of the ligaments and fractures of the bodies and pedicles of the vertebrae resulting in displacement of the vertebrae and loss of stability.

These are the fractures where the spinal cord is at considerable risk. If it is not damaged during the course of the displacement at the time of injury, it may be damaged by injudicious movement occurring after. FIRST AIDER: BE VERY CAREFUL WHEN TREATING THESE INJURIES OF THE SPINE.

Diagnosis

History. Careful questioning of the patient or bystanders may give important information as to how the injury was sustained. For example, the history may be of a car crash with a whiplash injury of the neck; diving into shallow water; the collapse of a rugby scrum; or being thrown from a motor cycle or horse. If the patient is unconscious with a head injury, particular attention must be paid to the neck, as injury to the cervical spine often accompanies head injuries. Therefore, if in any doubt, treat the unconscious patient as though he has a fracture of the cervical spine.

Symptoms and signs

General symptoms and signs. If there is a fracture of the cervical or thoracic spine with damage to the spinal cord, all the signs of shock will be present – pallor, cold clammy skin, rapid feeble pulse, and a lowered blood pressure.

Local symptoms and signs
1. Pain at the site of injury.
2. Referred pain around the body along the course of the nerve.
3. Tenderness.
4. Swelling with possible bruising.
5. Deformity, which may be marked with an abnormally prominent spinous process of the fractured vertebra, particularly noticeable in the thoracic spine.

   The skin may be very sensitive in a band around the body just above the site of the fracture. The spinal column above the site of injury tends to slide forward after the accident and compress the spinal cord, but it will also affect the nerve roots.

Injury to the spinal cord

There will be complete paralysis and loss of sensation below the level of the injury. The extent of the resulting paralysis will vary depending on the site of injury.

Cervical, or high, injuries will cause rapid death through paralysis of breathing.

Injuries below the 5th cervical vertebra will be associated with embarrassment of respiration because the only respiratory movement will be from the diaphragm. The thoracic muscles will not work. There will be complete paralysis of both arms and legs, i.e. quadriplegia.

With lower injuries there may be unusual movements of the arm because of unbalanced actions of those muscles that have escaped paralysis. The arms may be held in the 'hands up' position, for example.

In thoracic and lumbar injuries the upper limbs will escape damage but there will be paralysis of both lower limbs, while the abdominal muscles and viscera may be affected. Immediately after injury, acute retention of urine will develop because of inability to empty the bladder. Lumbar vertebral fractures may develop retroperitoneal bleeding followed by paralysis of the gut.

NECK INJURY

DO NOT MOVE

Listen

Pain
Funny feelings arms legs
Weakness arms legs

Look

Position held
Deformity

Feel gently

Pain? Deformity?

Immobilize

First aid treatment of spinal column injuries

If there is any doubt, all injuries of the spine must be treated as unstable fractures. Therefore everything must be done to protect the spinal cord from damage or further damage. The patient should be moved by stretcher in a very careful manner, and preferably transported on his back. **DO NOT MOVE THE PATIENT** until you have a proper stretcher. If necessary the football game must be stopped, even if it is the First Division; traffic must be stopped or diverted until the patient can be moved safely. Hasty movement might produce irreparable damage.

Immediate action. Warn the patient to lie absolutely still and send for an ambulance and doctor immediately. Cover the patient with blankets and maintain careful observation. If there is an associated head injury, ensure that the jaw is kept forward and there is no obstruction of respiration, e.g. by the tongue falling backwards.

Prepare the stretcher. A scoop-type stretcher is best (Fig. 22.4). It is firm, unyielding and can be placed under the patient without disturbing him unduly.

Failing this the canvas-type stretcher can be made more rigid by placing fracture boards across the framework. Cover the stretcher with a folded blanket and provide cushions to support the neck and small of the back when the patient is on the stretcher. Arrange the stretcher in line with the patient's body, with its head near his feet, since the patient is placed on this stretcher by firmly lifting the patient and placing the stretcher under him.

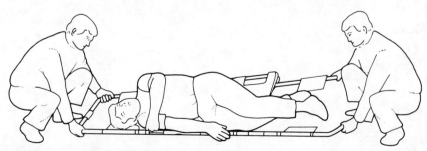

Fig. 22.4 Scoop stretcher. Courtesy of FW Equipment Co Ltd.

Prepare the patient. The patient must always be moved 'in one piece', that is by moving the body as a whole without disturbing the spine.

1. Place thin pads between the patient's thighs, knees and ankles, then tie both lower limbs together by broad bandages round the thighs and knees, and a narrow bandage as a figure-of-eight round the feet and ankles.

2. Instruct two assistants to apply gentle traction at the head and feet of the patient, respectively. Traction means gently pulling the part concerned and is similar in principle to extension of a limb, as is done for a fractured femur. Its object in the case of a fractured spine is to steady and support the vertebrae. Traction is undertaken as follows:

   (a) The assistant at the patient's head faces his feet, stoops down and places the palms of his hands on the patient's ears with his fingers at the back of the neck and his thumbs over the angles of the jaw. He gently draws the patient's head towards him, being careful not to raise it from the ground.

   (b) The assistant at the feet faces the patient's head, stoops down and with both hands grips the ankles from their outer sides. He applies traction keeping the feet on the ground. Traction must be maintained until the patient has been loaded on to the stretcher.

3. The patient has no sensation below the site of injury, so prevent damage to anaesthetic skin by emptying the patient's pockets where necessary.

Loading on to the stretcher – blanket method.

1. If the patient is lying in any position other than on his back, carefully roll him on to his back, on to a blanket if possible (Fig. 22.5), taking care to move his body as a whole and avoid twisting the spine. Make use of all available assistants for this purpose and have them move on your command.

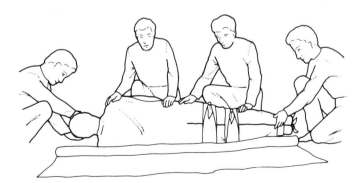

Fig. 22.5 The blanket method of lifting. The patient has been turned on to his left side by the bearers while the assistants are applying traction at the head and feet respectively. The two bearers who should be on the near side of the patient have been omitted for the sake of clarity. The rolled-up blanket is shown close to the patient's body.

2. The patient must now be placed on a blanket.
   (a) The blanket is rolled up lengthwise for half its width, and the roll placed close to the side of the patient's body.
   (b) While the assistants maintain traction, the bearers very carefully turn the patient on to his side, all helpers working together to move the body as a whole to prevent movement at the site of fracture.
   (c) The roll is placed close up to the side of the patient, who is then turned gently over the roll until he is lying on his opposite side.
   (d) The roll is now undone and the patient turned on to his back, so that he lies in the centre of the blanket.
   (e) If the patient was found on his side he should be rolled directly on to the blanket.
   (f) Each edge of the blanket is now rolled up firmly against the side of the patient's body.

Loading the stretcher – standard method. For satisfactory handling of the case, five assistants should be available, four to lift the patient (Fig. 22.6) and the other quickly to push the stretcher under him. This number of assistants is, of course, in addition to those applying traction. To facilitate description the assistants loading the stretcher are called bearers.

1. When lifting, the four bearers should arrange themselves in pairs facing each other on opposite sides of the patient's body.

2. They stoop and grasp the rolled edges of the blanket, with their hands fairly far apart.

3. At a given word of command, they gently rise, raising the patient with them to a height just sufficient to allow the fifth bearer to slip the stretcher under him. Just before this is done, the assistant applying traction at the feet must separate his legs widely to allow the stretcher to pass between them.

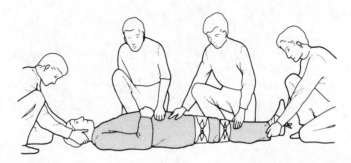

Fig. 22.6 Preparation for lifting. The two assistants are applying traction to the head and feet respectively and the two bearers shown are stooping in preparation for lifting. The two additional bearers on the near side of the patient have been omitted for the sake of clarity.

4. If only four bearers are available, they must arrange the stretcher as near to the patient as possible before lifting, and then move with short side-steps until the patient is over the stretcher and gently lower him on to it.

5. With only three bearers, two must lift and the third push the stretcher under the patient. Two bearers working alone must lift and carry the patient sideways on to the stretcher.

Emergency methods.

1. **Coat loading.** In the absence of a blanket the patient's clothing may be used to enable steady lifting. Traction is applied, the patient's coat is opened out and its edges rolled firmly inwards to make two improvised rolls, one on each side of his body. Loading is undertaken as before, the bearers not only grasping the coat but also the clothing or bandages round the patient's thighs. This is an alternative to the blanket method and only recommended for use as a substitute.

2. **Webbing bands.** These can be used when the above methods are unsuitable owing to debris or an uneven surface beneath the patient, or when his clothing is damaged or destroyed. They are worked under the body as follows:

    (a) the shoulders,

    (b) the small of the back,

    (c) the upper part of the thighs, and

    (d) the calves.

Four bearers arrange themselves as in the standard method and each grasp two handles, which are normally attached to the ends of the webbing bands. Head-end bearers hold those passing under the shoulders and thighs, while feet-end bearers grasp those from under the hips and calves. It will be noted that the middle handles cross each other.

Attention to head and neck. Support and traction of the head is necessary for all fractures except those in the lumbar region. In this case, the head need only be supported, while another assistant applies traction to the feet.

The Hines cervical splint is best used when extracting a trapped patient from a damaged car. Failing this, an improvised cervical splint (Fig. 22.7) can be made from a rolled newspaper and applied before moving the patient.

After care.

1. If the fracture is in the cervical region, a cervical splint should be applied. Place firm pads or sand bags on each side of the neck to prevent movement during transport.

. 2. Complete covering of the patient and continue simple care. Check that there are no objects between patient and stretcher likely to cause pressure.

3. If transport is over rough ground and likely to cause undue movement of

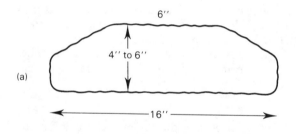

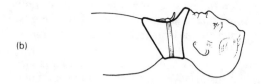

Fig. 22.7 Cervical collar: (a) rolled newspaper or doubled cardboard; (b) triangular bandage or scarf.

the patient on the stretcher, bind his body firmly but not tightly to the stretcher by broad bandages round the hips, thighs and calves.

4. On arrival at hospital do not unload the patient except on the instructions of a doctor.

Face downwards transport. This method is occasionally used, e.g. in coal mines, when the stretcher must not be boarded or when the patient has facial injuries.

Preparation of stretcher. The patient is to be transported in the prone position. Two blankets are folded in such a way that two-thirds of each blanket is placed on the stretcher, while the remaining third forms a flap stretching out from the side of the stretcher. There are thus four layers of blanket on the stretcher and two flaps, one on each side.

Two large pads are now made by folding and rolling two blankets. These pads must be firm and as wide as the stretcher.

Preparation of the patient

1. The lower limbs should be tied together as in the first method.
2. Three assistants should now carefully roll the patient on to his side and support him in this position. The body should be rolled as a whole. i.e. 'in one piece', so that no part of the spine is twisted.
3. The fourth assistant places the two pads in position, so that one pad rests on the front of the shoulders and the other across the front of the hips.
4. The stretcher, turned on its side, is now placed close up to the patient's body by the fourth assistant.

Lifting the patient on the stretcher. The four assistants, working in close cooperation, must now turn both patient and stretcher into the correct position for carrying. This involves turning patient and stretcher as if they were a single unit. It will be found during the process of turning that it is often necessary to lift the patient slightly, so that he is ultimately on the centre of the stretcher. The flaps are now folded over the patient's back to promote warmth, and his head turned slightly to one side and supported on a pillow for comfort.

Patient care. Whichever method is adopted, every effort must be made from the start to minimize the physical and mental stress of the injury by gentleness and confident reassurance.

— 23

Sports Injuries

With more people taking part in sport, more people are being injured. It is estimated that two million people a year suffer sports injuries, and 10% require time off work. Injuries may be either **acute**, due to trauma from a direct blow, twisting or falling; or **overuse injuries** following long periods of training (these are often aggravated by poor equipment or footwear). The injuries are very much the same as described under the various sections, but there are certain combinations of injuries which are frequently seen in specific types of sport.

It is at sports meetings the skilled first aider will be most in demand to deal with sports injuries (most of which are soft tissue injuries). The same principles apply as in all other injuries: the assessment of bruising, muscle strain, ligament sprain or bone fracture; history; examination; first aid treatment and referral to a hospital remain exactly the same.

Patterns of injury

Contact sports produce a large number of accidents, which are usually associated with direct or indirect trauma.

The martial arts, judo, karate and boxing involve injuries to the hand, shoulder, jaw, teeth, nose and brain (Fig. 23.1).

Association football produces injury to the lower limb, e.g. fractures of the tibia, fibula, the femur (occasionally), Potts' fractures, metatarsal fractures and frequently sprains of the ankle.

Rugby football. With different techniques of playing and tackling, injuries tend to occur to the upper limbs, with fracture of the clavicle or dislocation of the shoulder being particularly common. A more serious injury may be seen specifically when the scrum collapses. Injuries to the neck in rugby football must be treated seriously and regarded as a potential spinal fracture dislocation (see Chapter 22).

Cricket. Head and hand injuries are common, but the modern helmet protects the cranium and zygoma from injury. However, fractures of the fingers and metacarpals are relatively common (Fig. 23.2).

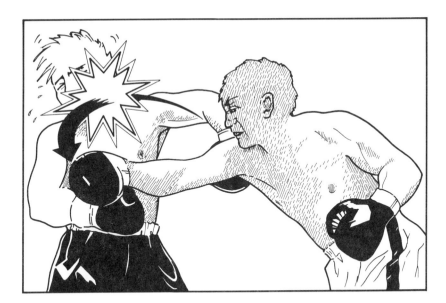

Fig. 23.1 Boxing injury.

Riding. The danger is when the horse throws the rider: head and spinal injuries are serious possibilities, although the B.S. 4472 jockey helmet offers far more protection than the old-fashioned riding hat. More frequently, dislocation of the shoulder or fracture of the clavicle will occur.

Parachuting. Injuries may occur during the exit or flight phase but are more common on landing, when the lower limb, and particularly the ankle, is at risk. If the parachute does not open properly more serious injuries to the spine or femur may occur. Concussion following injury to the head when landing backwards is seen on uncontrolled landings.

Common soft tissue injuries

Ligaments

Injuries to ligaments vary in degree, from sprain to rupture. With tearing of the fibres haemorrhage is followed by swelling and pain, and often with an effusion into the joint, so the patient is unable to use the joint.

On examination there is swelling around the joint and over the ligaments. The tenderness is on the ligament itself and not over the bone, enabling one

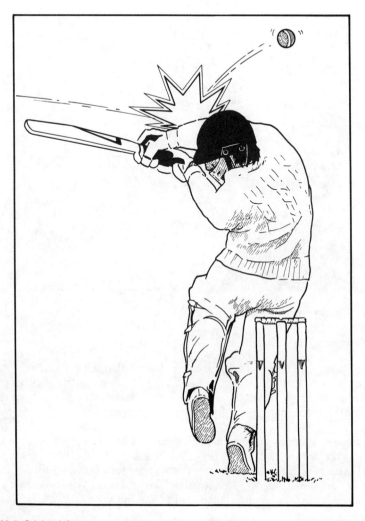

Fig. 23.2 Cricket injury.

to differentiate a sprain from a fracture. Movements are limited by the effusion and swelling.

Treatment

A cold compress, followed by a firm crepe bandage and elevation of the injured area, is important. With the common sprain, a combination of rest from weight-bearing accompanied by active exercise will enable the patient to return to sport and full activity much sooner. If there is any doubt about the presence of fracture, a medical opinion and an x-ray should be sought. Some of the joints most commonly involved are the following:

1. Ankle. The ligaments on the outside of the joint are most frequently involved, the anterior band being the most usually injured (Fig. 23.3). Swelling and tenderness occur anterior and inferior to the lateral malleolus. The middle band, below the tip of the lateral malleolus, is injured less frequently and generally only in connection with more serious injuries. If there is a complete tear to the ankle ligament, there is gross swelling and instability.

2. Knee. Ligament and capsular strain is common, but in addition there is the hazard of damage to the cartilages (the menisci) by excessive rotational strain on the knee. If swelling occurs immediately after the injury, it is suggestive of tearing of both the capsule and ligament. A gradual effusion, occurring 12–24 hours after the injury, is more suggestive of ligament or capsule sprain. Injuries to the menisci are associated with inability to move the joint; the knee locks and swells, and it is not possible to bend or straighten the joint.

Treatment. These injuries require a supporting bandage for treatment, and should be referred to a hospital for evaluation.

3. Shoulder joint. This is frequently sprained or dislocated. A dislocation implies tearing of the ligaments (see Chapter 21).

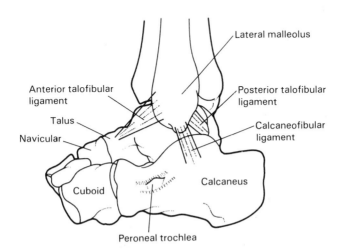

Fig. 23.3 Lateral side of left ankle joint.

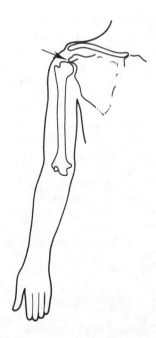

Fig. 23.4 Acromio-clavicular subluxation.

4. Acromioclavicular joint. This joint is frequently sprained following falls, with tenderness over the joint. The injury varies from a slightly tender, painful joint, to wide separation with elevation of the clavicle (Fig. 23.4). Differentiation from a fracture of the clavicle is often difficult. The arm should be placed in a triangular sling and an x-ray sought.

5. Thumb. Injuries to the metacarpophalangeal joint of the thumb (Fig. 23.5) occur frequently in skiing and polo, and are known as 'gamekeeper's thumb'. There is tearing of the ligament on the inner side of the thumb, with instability and a weak grip. In cases of a complete tear as opposed to a sprain, operative treatment is required to restore the stability of the joint.

Muscle injury

Muscle injuries are common, particularly at the beginning of the season when adequate training has not been carried out and excessive strain occurs. If the patient has not had the chance to warm up, there is greater danger. Muscles most commonly damaged are those in the thigh (the rectus femoris), behind the knee (the hamstring), and in the groin (the adductor). In the calf, the calf muscles and Achilles tendon are frequently damaged, particularly in tennis and squash. A muscle tear is followed by a haematoma which becomes hard and fibrotic.

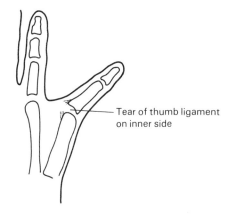
Tear of thumb ligament
on inner side

Fig. 23.5 Gamekeeper's thumb.

Treatment

Application of cold compresses or ice, followed by firm bandaging to prevent excessive swelling, and early exercise (without bearing weight on the injured part) should be encouraged. If there is severe bruising, medical treatment should be sought, as often fibrosis, with shortening, may occur in muscles.

Minor injuries of feet

Blisters. These are common early in the season or when the patient is using a new pair of shoes. Clean the blisters and surrounding area well with spirit, drain the blister, apply an antiseptic and cover with a sticking plaster or other adhesive dressing. The feet should then be attended to, using foot powder, and clean socks which fit and not forgetting to ease the training shoes.

Acute foot strain is often seen at the beginning of the season, the result of running too far too soon. Initially, rest and hot-and-cold contrast foot-baths are recommended followed by gently progressive activity, ensuring that the patient is wearing comfortable footwear.

Overuse injuries in training

A poor training schedule with repetitive minor trauma will lead to chronic injury and strain. Good equipment, particularly footwear, is essential for training as well as for the event itself.

Achilles tendonitis. There is thickening and tenderness over the body of the Achilles tendon. This·can be made worse by a shoe with a high back.

Treatment. The foot should be rested, and pressure on the tendon avoided. A shoe with a slightly higher heel should be used or a Sorbothane® heel cushion inserted. This takes a lot of the pressure away from the heel.

Muscle injury. With heavy training schedules, especially when running on roads, there is a long series of jarring shocks through the legs. A lot of repetitive movements take place at a steady pace and speed. Overtraining injures the hamstring and calf muscles. A sudden increase in activity, or in the stride, can produce a muscle tear.

Treatment. Often by changing the training schedule, using different shoes and a Sorbothane® heel pad, this condition will be relieved. Rest followed by contrast baths and physiotherapy may be required for extreme cases.

Stress fractures. The recurrent trauma of hard training can produce small cracks in the bone. These are stress fractures (Fig. 23.6), and commonly occur in the leg, e.g. the fibula, the tibia, occasionally the neck of femur, and commonly on the second or third metatarsal bones of the foot. There is a history of increasing intensity in training over several weeks, followed by pain and tenderness occurring for two to three weeks.

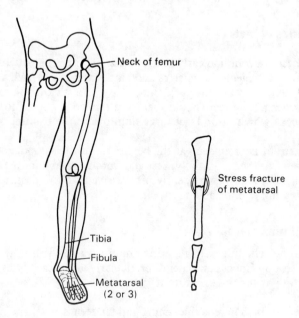

Fig. 23.6 Stress fractures.

Treatment is rest for 4–6 weeks. If this condition is suspected the patient should be seen by a doctor, as the diagnosis can only be confirmed by x-rays, which often have to be repeated.

Jogger's nipple. Running for several hours in the rain, or while sweating heavily, may produce a sore bleeding nipple if the vest or shirt is tight (Fig. 23.7). The nipple should be protected by an adhesive dressing and a looser shirt worn.

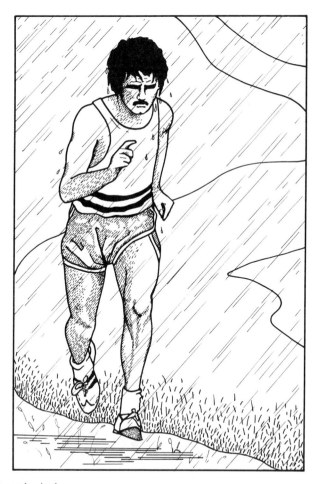

Fig. 23.7 Jogger's nipple.

Shin soreness

Shin splints: after excessive training there is a tender area over the shin. This is probably the pulling off of muscle fibres from the bone, but it may be the early stage of a stress fracture. If pain does not settle after rest, a doctor should be consulted.

Compartment syndrome: the leg has a strong envelope of fascia. If the bulk of the shin muscle increases considerably in a short time, e.g. during training, extra activity, such as running, will produce pain. Treatment is to rest the limb.

Marathon running and jogging. These activities are becoming much more popular, and hundreds of thousands of people are participating. In the first aid arrangements for these events, attention should be paid to the acute and overuse injuries already described. Unaccustomed exercise in the middle-aged may produce angina or heart attacks. Long runs in bad weather conditions produce their own problems, particularly in the unfit. In hot weather, which induces excess sweating, there is a danger of heat exhaustion. In conditions of high humidity and low air movement, heat stroke is possible. Cold, wet weather, with the wind producing a chill factor, will increase the dangers of hypothermia. Special precautions need to be taken, e.g. refreshment points and first aid stations at frequent intervals.

— 24

Unconsciousness – General Principles

Unconsciousness is a serious state, so the patient's condition may cause anxiety and worry to the first aider. However, prompt, efficient action which secures a good airway and removes any obstruction such as blood, vomit or dentures may prevent complications and save the life of the patient.

The causes of loss of consciousness are numerous, the common ones only will be described.

Primary causes

The patient becomes unconscious as the immediate result of any injury or a disease affecting the central nervous system.

Head injuries

1. Concussion.
2. Contusion.
3. Laceration.
4. Compression of the brain.

Medical diseases

1. Stroke.
2. Epileptic fits.
3. Infantile convulsions.

Psychogenic (hysteria etc.)

The patients are not truly unconscious but **appear** unconscious.

Poisoning

1. Narcotics.
2. Alcohol or drugs.
3. Effects of current drug therapy overdose (blood pressure and heart, diabetes, nerves, steroids).

Secondary causes

Complications from an injury or disease affecting other systems of the body involve the nervous system, producing unconsciousness.
1. Asphyxia.
2. Oxygen lack (hypoxia).
3. Fainting (syncope).
4. Heart attack.
5. Diabetic coma (hyperglycaemia) or hypoglycaemia.
6. Kidney disease (uraemia).
7. Heat illness.

Method of investigation

History

If the cause is obvious (e.g. epilepsy) or where immediate treatment for asphyxia is essential, treatment must be started before taking the history. Usually, however, a careful history is required and should be obtained from bystanders or relatives if possible. The following points need clarification:

Possibility of injury. Was the patient injured before becoming unconscious?

Mode of onset. Was the loss of consciousness gradual or sudden? A gradual onset suggests the possibility of poisoning or alcohol, but also occurs occasionally in compression of the brain or stroke.

Previous attacks. Similar attacks occurring previously, especially if it is epilepsy or hysteria, give important clues to diagnosis. Hysteria, however, should be diagnosed with caution as important medical conditions may be missed.

Former health. A history of diabetes or kidney disease can possibly be obtained.

A special bracelet or card may be carried by the patient, particularly heart patients, diabetics, epileptics or patients receiving steroids. Bottles containing tablets or poisons may be found.

Examination

A quick first aid assessment and examination should be made, checking the airway, whether or not there is bleeding, the state of the chest and abdomen and whether fractures of the limbs are present.

Special physical signs

Depth of unconsciousness. It is important that the level of consciousness is noted and timed. If there is any change in the level of consciousness, this must be noted and the time recorded.

The levels described merge one into the other and there may be slow or rapid movement from one level to another. All these are of significance in establishing a diagnosis or assessing progress of the patient.

1. Lucid. The patient is cooperative and conscious.
2. Confusion. He is disorganized but will obey commands.
3. Semi-coma. The patient will only react to painful stimuli but not voice commands; unconscious.
4. Coma. There is no response to stimuli; deeply unconscious.

Glasgow Coma Scale. This scale is widely accepted in hospitals and is an easily understood description of the level of consciousness. It gets rid of the vague expressions which have been used for many years to describe unconscious people. This scale (see Table 24.1) should always be used.

Respiration. The breathing may be quick, shallow, stertorous (snoring) or irregular. Stertorous breathing tends to occur in deeper unconsciousness

Table 24.1 Glasgow Coma Scale.

Eyes open	– Spontaneously – To speech – To pain – None (no opening)	All self-evident, not a good indicator of conscious level alone.
***Best* verbal response**		
Orientated	– Knows name, place, year, season and month.	
Confused conversation	– Attention held, conversational response, but disorientated and confused.	
Inappropriate words	– Intelligible articulation, non-conversational, abusive or swear words.	
Incomprehensible sounds	– Moans and groans, no recognizable words.	
None	– None.	
***Best* motor response**	– Best arm response usually recorded, do not misinterpret reflex grasping.	
Obeys commands	– Best response. If negative use painful stimulus.	
Localize pain	– Causes the limb to move in an attempt to remove the stimulus.	
Flexion to pain	– Can vary in degree.	
Extension to pain	– U.L.: Arm adducted and extended at elbow, forearm pronated. – L.L.: Extension at hip and knee, plantar flexion of foot.	
None	– None.	

(coma) and may also be seen in stroke, epilepsy or severe head injuries, and in some cases of poisoning. Irregular breathing, particularly if there are short periods when breathing stops, is a bad sign. It may occur after severe head injury, poisoning or uraemia.

Eyes. Examination of the eyes and the pupils and their reaction to light is always of great value in establishing the diagnosis.

Pupil size. The pupils may be small (contracted) or large (dilated). They may be equal or unequal. Contracted pupils may indicate poisoning e.g. from heroin or other opiates, while inequality of the pupils usually suggests compression of the brain or stroke. Dilated pupils may result from atropine (belladonna) ingestion, cerebral hypoxia or other brain stem damage.

Pupil reaction. The pupils normally become smaller when exposed to light. This reaction is seen when raising the eyelids or shining a light into the eyes, when the pupils will become smaller. The light response may be absent in coma or poisoning from narcotics.

The pulse rate must be noted. A rapid pulse occurs in shock, fainting, collapse and sometimes concussion of the brain. A slow pulse may result from stroke or cerebral compression. Irregularity of the pulse occurs in diseases affecting the heart, and also in the later stages of poisoning.

Odour of breath. The odour of the breath should be carefully noted, as it may supply a clue in a case of poisoning. The smell of alcohol should be noted but does not always indicate a diagnosis of drunkenness. The patient may have taken alcohol because he felt ill, or may have had a head injury or stroke after having a drink. **Drunkenness should be regarded as the last diagnosis in unconscious patients.** Other factors, most notably a low blood sugar (hypoglycaemia), must always be excluded. In uraemia the breath may smell rather like urine, whilst in diabetes a faint aroma of acetone or nail varnish may be noticed.

Convulsions are violent, irregular movements of the limbs or body caused by involuntary muscular action. Convulsions occur in epilepsy, uraemia, and sometimes in hypertension. Twitchings may precede infantile (febrile) convulsions.

Paralysis. Paralysis is the loss of muscle power and is usually due to disease of the nervous system. It occurs commonly after a stroke or cerebral compression. It can be recognized by the presence of limpness affecting one side of the body.

Limb movement. First three sections refer to voluntary movement, last three the response to painful stimuli.
1. Normal power – Self-evident.
2. Mild weakness – Can move the limb against gravity.
3. Severe weakness – Flicker movement to power unable to overcome gravity.
4. Spastic flexion – Shoulder abduction, elbow flexion, hand closed, increased tone.
5. Extension – Extensor response to painful stimulus.
6. No response – No response.

Fits. If fits occur record details.

Incontinence. Patients sometimes pass urine or defaecate involuntarily. This is incontinence and may occur in epilepsy, infantile convulsions and stroke. Unconsciousness may be profound, resulting in the patient losing full control of his bowels.

Rigidity. The muscles become stiff and firm and cannot be relaxed by the patient. It is a form of muscle spasm. Rigidity may affect the whole body in cases of epilepsy, tetanus and strychnine poisoning, or only specific groups of muscles may be involved. After a partial fracture of the spine, localized rigidity may be found in the overlying muscles.

Principles of treatment

First aid treatment must often start before the diagnosis has been made.

Life saving measures: airway, breathing, and circulation. Bleeding or cardiac arrest must be treated immediately after triage. It cannot be emphasized often enough that the airways of unconscious patients must be cleared of blood, vomit, and/or dentures to avoid further damage to the brain by asphyxia.

Position. Whatever the cause of the unconsciousness, the patient must be placed in the recovery position with the body sloping head down. If on a stretcher or bed, the foot should be raised.

Medical aid. An ambulance or doctor should be sent for immediately. All tight clothing around the neck, chest and waist should be loosened to improve breathing.

Warmth. A blanket should be used to prevent the patient becoming cold.

Space. Bystanders should be prevented from crowding round the patient and windows and doors opened to supply adequate fresh air if the room is too hot.

Removal. The patient should be moved to shelter from the elements or from dangerous positions after the life saving measures have been carried out.

Fluids. No food or drink should ever be given by mouth to unconscious patients. This includes whisky or brandy. After the patient has recovered consciousness he may request a drink, in which case a few sips of water may be given. However, if the patient has an injury which requires surgery, no fluid should be given.

Observation. An unconscious patient should never be left unattended. He should be carefully watched after he returns to consciousness.

Death

The diagnosis of death is often difficult even for a doctor. Modern methods of cardiopulmonary resuscitation have often restored life after breathing has ceased and the pulse has apparently disappeared. It is therefore important that resuscitation is started and continued until a medical opinion has been obtained. The feelings of relatives and friends must be respected.

Signs of death

Colour and expression. The normal colour of the patient disappears and is replaced by a greyish hue. The expression on the face changes and becomes inanimate.

Cooling. The temperature of the body falls rapidly when death occurs.

Eyes. The eyeball loses its firmness when touched through the eyelid with the finger; the eyes themselves lose their lustre and the pupils are dilated and do not react to light.

Limpness. All the muscles of the body become loose and the jaw usually drops, thus opening the mouth. In the course of six hours or so the muscles gradually become stiff as rigor mortis sets in.

— 25 ——————————————————

Head, Brain and Facial Injury

Injuries to the head and brain are common in contact sports (such as boxing), assaults and road traffic accidents. High speed motorcycle or motorcar accidents are likely to cause more severe injuries. However, comparatively minor blows can fracture the skull and, if followed by bleeding, may cause cerebral compression. Any patient who has had a head injury producing unconsciousness should be seen by a doctor.

Trauma can result in:

(a) scalp injury,
(b) brain injury,
(c) fractured skull, or
(d) facial injuries.

SCALP INJURY

The scalp is thick skin, firmly attached to a layer of fibrous tissue (the aponeurosis) which extends over the vault of the skull (Fig. 25.1). Beneath the aponeurosis is a layer of loose connective tissue, covering the pericranium, which is firmly attached to the bones of the skull. This loose layer is responsible for the ease with which the scalp can be detached by injury.

It has a rich blood and nerve supply. Numerous veins pass from the scalp to the venous sinuses within the skull, providing a portal of entry for infection. Infection may cause infection of the bone (osteomyelitis) or, if it

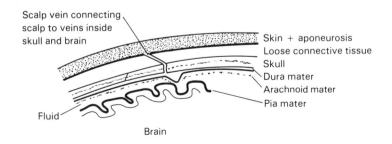

Fig. 25.1 Scalp, skull, lining membranes and brain.

spreads into the brain, may cause meningitis or even cerebral abscess. This is why all lacerations of the scalp must be treated with great care.

Because of the rich blood supply, wounds of the scalp bleed profusely, and often this bleeding will not stop until the scalp is firmly sutured. Sometimes, following a blow, a haematoma will form in the skin or under the scalp. This swelling will be seen soon after the injury.

Treatment of scalp lacerations

The hair around the edge of the wound will require cutting with scissors, and the skin should then be carefully washed with antiseptic solution. Dirt should be gently washed away from the wound, but any foreign body embedded in the wound should be left in situ. Bleeding should be controlled by a firm pad and bandage. If there is a protruding foreign body, surround this with a ring bandage to avoid applying pressure to the foreign body. Further treatment will be required in the A & E Department of the nearest hospital.

BRAIN INJURY

Most injuries to the head are associated with a moving force, and it is the effect of this force on the brain which is responsible for the damage (Fig. 25.2). Acceleration or deceleration injuries will cause a shearing stress in the brain tissues. There is displacement or distortion of brain tissue at the time of impact, particularly in deceleration, e.g. when a motorcyclist is thrown and his head hits the ground. The acceleration type of injury occurs due to blows from boxing or assault. The injury to the brain may vary in degree from concussion to coma: this will depend on the amount of stretch and displacement of the brain substance and the cumulative damage to the brain cells.

Effect on the brain

The effect of applied force is to interfere with consciousness. For ease of description, certain levels of consciousness are defined. These levels, however, merge gradually into one another, and movement between them can occur slowly or rapidly.

1. Lucid – the patient is cooperative: conscious.
2. Confusion – he is disorientated but will obey commands.
3. Semi-coma – the patient will react to painful stimuli but not to voice commands: unconscious.
4. Coma – there is no response to stimuli: deeply unconscious.

   Depending on the severity of injury, there may be loss of memory of events occurring before the accident (retrograde amnesia). There may also be

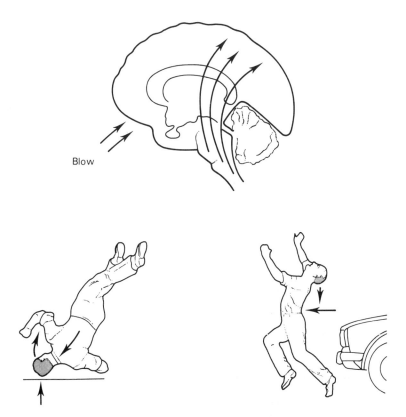

Fig. 25.2 Shearing force acting on the brain.

loss of memory for things occurring after the accident (post-traumatic amnesia). The length of time of these periods of amnesia is a very good indication of the amount of damage the patient's brain has sustained.

Contusion

The damage to the brain tissue ruptures the nerve fibres. There may be movement between the grey matter and the white matter of the brain. The period of unconsciousness is more prolonged, and recovery is usually slower. Contusion is often associated with bruising and oedema, and with areas of damaged brain cells. The patient passes from a state of confusion into a state of cerebral irritability. The patient is initially pale, with shallow respirations, increased pulse rate and relaxed muscles. If the damage is more severe the respirations become deeper. On recovery, during the stage of cerebral irritability, there may be resentment, and the patient may curl up away from the light. Afterwards there may be minor personality changes and interference with memory, which should improve with time.

Laceration and brain stem damage

The damage to the brain tissue in these cases is more severe than in contusion; there is tearing in addition to the bruising and bleeding. The patient is in a deep coma and does not respond to stimuli. The pupils are dilated, the pulse is irregular and the respiration periodically ceases for short intervals. This is called 'Cheyne–Stokes respiration'. Recovery is slow, and often the patient is left with signs of permanent brain damage.

Brain compression

Blood accumulating either
 (a) between the dura and the skull,
 (b) between the meninges and the brain, or
 (c) in the brain itself,
will cause a rise in intracranial pressure (Fig. 25.3). Often, after a period of unconsciousness, the patient recovers and his mind is quite clear – this is the lucid interval. He then develops a headache which becomes more severe; he may start vomiting. The level of consciousness gradually deteriorates from lucid to confusion to semi-coma to coma. When he is semi-comatose, there is increased restlessness and he only responds to painful stimuli. The pupils will change in size and their reaction to light will cease. Initially, the pupil on the same side as the brain compression increases in size and then does not react to light. As the pressure increases, the pupil on the other side also increases in size. This is why it is so important to register the size of the pupil and the

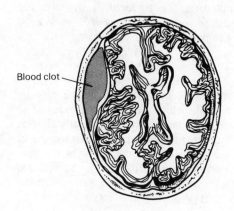

Blood clot

Fig. 25.3 Haemorrhage within the skull. Note how the brain is being compressed.

time, so that the doctor may assess how quickly the compression is developing. As the level of consciousness descends, the muscles on the other side of the body become weaker, so it is important to note the power of the muscles as well.

Post-head injury problems

The rate of recovery from a head injury depends on the degree of damage to the brain. Transient loss of consciousness, lasting from a few seconds to several weeks, may occur. The patient may complain of headaches and vaguely feeling off-colour after minor head injury, but this will improve.

After severe contusion or laceration with actual brain damage, recovery is much slower. Apart from interference with limb movements there may be personality changes. These may cause situations in which the first aider may be involved, so it is best he should know of the possibility. The patient may become aggressive and tires quickly. He finds it difficult to concentrate and notices that his memory is not as good as it was. This condition will improve with time, but recovery is slow, from 18–24 months.

Examination of a patient with a head injury

It is most important that observations are made by the skilled first aider on first seeing the patient. It is a good idea to write these down and note the times, so that when the patient is taken to the A & E Department there is a record of the early physical signs. These will be of great importance for assessing the treatment required.

History

Often it may be important to act quickly to clear the patient's airway before speaking to onlookers, but at some stage find out exactly what happened to the patient – what type of accident took place, and whether the patient was initially unconscious or not. How long had he been unconscious, and when did he recover consciousness? Had there been significant blood loss, and had any drink been taken? There may be relatives or friends present who can give details of his previous medical history.

The patient may also be carrying a special card or bracelet which warns of his being a diabetic or epileptic, or that he is taking special drugs or steroids.

Examination of patient

Airway. The first thing to do is to make sure that the patient's airway is clear. Much of the brain damage from head injuries is the result of a poor air supply due to vomit, blood clot or dentures impacted in the back of the mouth. If any of these is inhaled into the lungs, more serious damage occurs.

General examination. A quick examination of the whole body should be made at this stage, noting any fractures or other injuries. The head should be inspected for lacerations, bruising or puffiness suggestive of an underlying fracture, bleeding from the ears or nose, or the loss of a clear fluid (cerebrospinal fluid) through the nose. Assess other injuries, including those to the face and the neck. Injuries to the cervical spine often occur at the same time as head injury. In road traffic accidents the chest, abdomen, spine and limbs should also be quickly assessed for signs of damage.

Level of consciousness. It is important to record the time and note the level of consciousness: this is most effectively done according to the modern method known as the 'Glasgow Coma Scale' (Fig. 25.4). This shows the functional level of consciousness, and the terms are used in all hospital accident departments so that comparisons can be drawn.

If there is any change in any of these observations, it should be noted along with the time it took place.

Pupils. An assessment of the size of the pupils should be made. Are they of equal size or is one dilated? Do they react to light during examination? Do

		Date:
		Time
C O M A S C A L E	EYES OPEN (Eyes closed by swelling = C)	Spontaneously To speech To pain None
	BEST VERBAL RESPONSE	Orientated Confused Inappropriate words Incomprehensible sounds None
	BEST MOTOR RESPONSE (Better arm)	Obey commands Localise pain Flexion to pain Extension to pain None

Fig. 25.4 Glasgow Coma Scale.

PUPILS	R	Size	$\left(\begin{array}{c}+\\\text{or}\\-\end{array}\right)$
(C = eye closed)		Reaction	
	L	Size	$\left(\begin{array}{c}+\\\text{or}\\-\end{array}\right)$
		Reaction	

Fig. 25.5 Recording of pupil size and reaction.

they contract easily or are they fixed (Fig. 25.5)? This information is recorded together with the time. It is sometimes easier to draw the size of the pupil (Fig. 25.6): this also makes it easier for comparisons to be made.

Limb movements. If possible an assessment of limb movements is made according to the chart (Fig. 25.7), and again these are recorded, together with the time of observation. What the observer is looking for is any change from a normal limb with normal power, through several stages of weakness or rigidity (spasticity) in both arms and legs.

Treatment

The patient should be placed in the recovery position. As emphasized at the beginning of this section it is important that the airway is cleared, that any blood, vomit or dentures are cleared from the mouth. It is important that fluids should not be given, as there is considerable danger of aspiration.

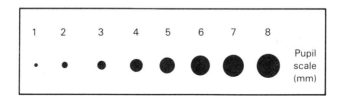

| 1 | 2 | 3 | 4 | 5 | 6 | 7 | 8 | Pupil scale (mm) |

Fig. 25.6 Size of pupil.

L I M B	A R M S	Normal power
M O V E M E N T		Mild weakness
		Severe weakness
		Spastic flexion
		Extension
		No response
	L E G S	Normal power
		Mild weakness
		Severe weakness
		Extension
		No response

Fig. 25.7 Limb movements.

If there are injuries of the limbs the patient is better placed lying on the side of the fractures. Suitable splintage should be carried out for fractures.

Repeated observations should be carried out and recorded.

Complications

Cerebral compression developing from a blood clot (haematoma) within the skull is a dangerous possibility.

Extradural haematoma. This complication typically follows the pattern of a head injury with unconsciousness, followed by a return of consciousness; the patient may feel quite well. After this lucid interval, the patient's condition deteriorates (with headache and vomiting) until he becomes semi-comatose, then comatose, and finally may die from cerebral compression. This usually occurs within the first 24 hours after the injury. The patient's level of consciousness changes – the pulse rate becomes slower, the pupils dilate, firstly on the side of the injury and later on the other side. **If, following a head injury, a patient has lost consciousness and then becomes restless with headaches, or if there is any deterioration in his level of consciousness, he must be taken to an A & E Department urgently.** Be aware of the unconscious man who smells of alcohol – he may not be drunk; he may have a head injury with developing cerebral compression. If in doubt take him to the hospital, as he may have a fractured skull with a tear in the middle meningeal artery.

Subdural haematoma. This complication tends to occur in older people. It often follows a trivial injury with movement of the brain in the skull. Small veins from the brain to the venous sinuses are torn, and the resultant blood clot develops slowly over a period of days or weeks. The initial injury is often so trivial that it is forgotten.

The typical history is from a patient over 50 who develops recurrent headaches of increasing severity, associated with drowsiness, apathy and confusion. Response to questions is slow and eventually the patient becomes stuporous. Recurrent symptoms of this nature should be investigated by a doctor.

FRACTURES OF THE SKULL

It is obvious that the most important factor in head injury is damage to the brain, with disturbances in the level of consciousness. It is the 'chocolates within the chocolate box' which are important. However, bony injury to the skull should also be understood, as this is so often associated with brain damage.

Fractures of the vault of the skull

These may vary from a small indentation (a depressed fracture) to gross fractures as seen following severe motorcycle accidents. The depressed fracture (Fig. 25.8) occurring after a blow with a blunt instrument is often an 'open' one. Penetrating fractures resulting from a gunshot wound, fragments of an exploding bomb, or the common dart, are often associated with little disturbance of consciousness. The wound should be treated by a sterile dressing and the patient placed in the recovery position. The penetrating foreign body, if protruding, must not be removed, but must be prevented from causing further damge, e.g. by placing a ring bandage around it and a dressing over the top.

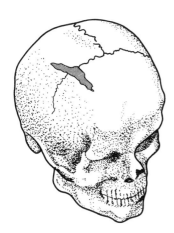

Fig. 25.8 Depressed fracture of the skull. Note: the fragment has been forced inwards towards the brain.

Fractures of the base of the skull

These occur after severe compression and deforming injuries. They are frequently seen as a result of road traffic accidents. The fracture line extends along the base of the skull (Fig. 25.9), and may interfere with nerves passing through various openings in the base.

Fractures of the anterior (front) fossa often discharge blood or clear cerebrospinal fluid through the nose. Bleeding can extend into the back of the eye, passing forward over the white of the eyeball. Fractures of the middle fossa will often interfere with the nerve of hearing or the motor nerve to the face, and there is bleeding from the ear. Rarely, the posterior (back) fossa of the skull is fractured; the back of the head feels 'boggy', with a swelling over the occiput (Fig. 25.10). Basal fractures often involve the air sinuses and are technically 'open' from within.

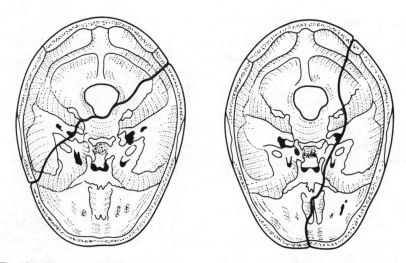

Fig. 25.9 Fractures of the base of the skull. The thick lines represent sites of fractures.

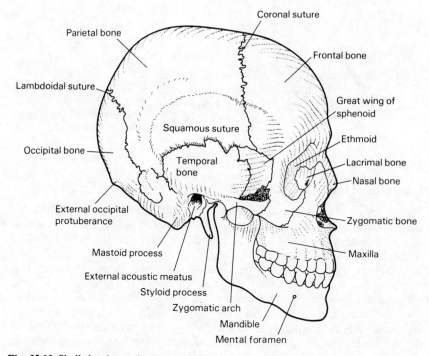

Fig. 25.10 Skull showing occiput, vault and base.

INJURIES OF THE FACE

The skin of the face, like that of the scalp, has a very good blood and nerve supply. Lacerations bleed heavily, but because of this rich blood supply they also heal rapidly. Wounds associated with gunshot or fragments from bombs appear gross, but early surgery is most effective.

The dangers from facial injury are the inhalation of blood and the state of consciousness of the patient. It is important that the airway is kept clear, and if the wound involves the nose and mouth, that the patient is treated in the recovery position so that saliva and blood can run out of the mouth and not be inhaled. Wounds should be dressed with a sterile pad and bandage. The patient must be evacuated in the recovery position and kept under observation.

Fracture of the nose

This is a very common injury and results in bleeding, obstruction to the nasal airway, and deformity. Bleeding often stops spontaneously, but the airway obstruction and deformity require assessment in a hospital.

Fractures of the maxilla

These vary from small alveolar fractures, involving one or two teeth, to a gross fracture of the facial skeleton where the whole of the maxilla is pushed backwards by a heavy blow. The significant factors are the state of consciousness and the risk of inhalation of blood or vomit. Often the injury is not apparent because the face rapidly swells from oedema and bruising, and it is only with x-rays that the amount of displacement can be assessed. If the fracture involves only one side of the maxilla, there is often interference with the sensations of the cheek, the gum and the teeth on that side.

Fracture of the zygoma

This is common after a blow from a fist or a cricket ball. It may cause double vision because of the alteration in the level of the floor of the orbit. Again, this is only obvious during the first half hour after the accident, because the cheek bruises and rapidly swells. The bone deformity is less obvious, and this is only apparent after 7–10 days, when the swelling has settled. This injury is often associated with difficulty in opening the mouth. Early hospital assessment and x-rays are required.

Fractures of the lower jaw (the mandible)

History

This fracture is common after a blow on the jaw (Fig. 25.11). The fracture may involve the horizontal or the ascending ramus, or the condyle of the mandible.

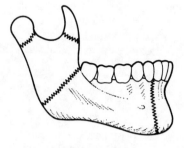

Fig. 25.11 Fractures of the jaw: commonest sites of occurrence.

Symptoms and signs

The patient will often support the fractured jaw with the palm of his hand. He complains of difficulty in opening the jaw, or pain on chewing, after a blow. There is tenderness over the site of the fracture of the mandible and pain on opening the mouth. The teeth are irregular. As these are often open fractures, bleeding occurs from the gum, staining the saliva. In severe cases, if there is comminution or bilateral fracture of the jaw, control of the tongue is lost, and this may fall backwards causing interference with respiration: the patient must be transported prone (Fig. 25.12).

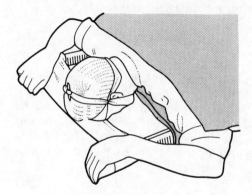

Fig. 25.12 Transport when both sides of lower jaw are fractured.

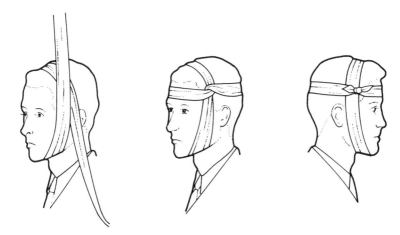

Fig. 25.13 Treatment of fracture of the jaw.

Treatment

1. The patient should sit down, leaning slightly forward supporting his jaw.
2. A pad is placed under the jaw, and the irregularity of the lower teeth is gently corrected by pressure against the upper jaw (Fig. 25.13).
3. Place the centre of a narrow bandage under the chin. Carry one end over the top of the head and cross it with the other above the ear. This leaves one end short and the other long.
4. Take the long end round the back of the skull and the shorter end round the forehead just above the eyebrows, tying the ends above the opposite ear.
5. Note: if the bandage is too short, tie over the top of the head as far forwards as possible. Another narrow bandage can be tied horizontally around the forehead, looping around the vertical bandages.

26

Medical Causes of Unconsciousness

EPILEPSY

Epilepsy is a disease of the nervous system, which is characterized by sudden attacks of unconsciousness known as fits. Two varieties of this complaint occur – major epilepsy (grand mal), in which the attacks of unconsciousness are accompanied by convulsions, and minor epilepsy (petit mal) in which convulsions are absent.

The disease usually begins in early adult life and fits may occur at intervals, depending upon the severity of the case. Thus, in slight forms of the disease, only one or two fits occur during the course of a year, but in more serious cases fits may recur at short intervals. In severe cases, there may be a sequence of convulsions without regaining consciousness. This is known as 'status epilepticus'. Fortunately, doctors can prescribe a combination of drugs which can prevent the occurrence of attacks.

Major epilepsy

A patient who is about to have an epileptic fit often experiences a warning, known as the 'aura', which calls his attention to the fact that an attack is imminent. This warning may provide him with an opportunity of placing himself in a position of safety before he is overcome by unconsciousness.

This aura takes the form of some subjective sensory premonition, such as numbness, giddiness or even a certain smell, which warns the patient that a fit is imminent.

Soon after the aura the patient may utter a shrill cry and drop to the ground, sometimes hurting himself severely through his fall. He is now immediately and completely unconscious and passes into the first stage of the fit, known as rigidity (tonic phase). Alternatively, the fit may commence with gradual twitching in one part of the body, which spreads until the whole body twitches (clonic phase) and the patient lies unconscious.

Rigidity

The patient lies on the ground, absolutely stiff, his fists clenched and all his muscles rigid, so that it is impossible to bend his arms or legs. The teeth are firmly clenched and the mouth cannot be opened. The muscles of respiration

230

are similarly in a state of spasm, and thus the patient is unable to breathe; for this reason his colour changes rapidly. He is at first pale, but quickly becomes blue (cyanosed).

The eyes may remain open and turned to one side; moreover, owing to the temporary cessation of respiration with contracted muscles, the whites of the eyes become red and congested.

The patient exhibits a pitiful appearance at this stage, and just as it would appear that he is on the verge of death, twitchings begin in his body as the attack passes into the stage of convulsions.

Convulsions

Forcible and involuntary muscular contractions now involve all the muscles in the body. The convulsions extend to the muscles of the jaw, and the saliva in the mouth is beaten up into a foam. Moreover, the tongue and cheeks are frequently bitten, thus blood-stained froth may be seen escaping from the lips.

The face next assumes a purplish colour, and the eyeballs appear to be protruding from their sockets. Urine and faeces may be passed involuntarily. This stage lasts from two to three minutes, but breathing, though jerky, prevents death by asphyxia. The convulsions gradually pass off and the breathing becomes easier.

Consciousness may quickly be recovered, and the patient is left pale, sweating, and exhausted. He shows little interest in his surroundings and may express the desire for sleep, a tendency which should be encouraged. Sometimes, however, consciousness is not recovered immediately, and the patient gradually passes into a condition of coma, consisting of deep unconsciousness accompanied by stertorous breathing. Coma gradually passes into a natural sleep, from which the patient finally awakes.

Treatment

An epileptic fit is a very unpleasant sight to witness and the first aider must not be alarmed by the appearance of the patient. Fortunately, death in an attack is extremely rare, and a competent first aider can do much for the patient at this stage. It is important, however, to reassure relatives and bystanders who may be present that the fit will quickly pass off and the patient recover. Treatment of a fit can be considered under its respective stages as follows:

Stage of rigidity

The most important first aid measure is to ensure that the patient does not further injure himself. He should be able to lie flat and all objects be removed from his vicinity.

Airway. If the patient can be supported on his side, this will be of value in maintaining his airway. It will not be possible to force open the patient's jaw, and forcing a gag between the teeth is undesirable at this stage.

Clothing. Undo tight clothing round the neck, chest and waist.

Space. Keep back bystanders. It must be remembered, however, that the stage of rigidity only lasts about half a minute, so there is not much time available for treatment (or indeed a need for it).

Stage of convulsions

Apply gag. The patient's jaw will relax slightly; this may allow a protective gag to be placed between the teeth to prevent further biting of the tongue. The gag should be a firm object which has been wrapped in some soft material, e.g. a handkerchief. The airway should be maintained by clearing any debris or false teeth from the mouth if possible, and supporting the patient on his side.

Sources of danger. Continue to ensure that all objects and persons are clear of the patient's limbs, to prevent further injury.

Support. Support the head to prevent from injury, and if possible support the patient on his side, but **in no way try to control** the convulsions.

Stage of recovery

Examination. A quick examination of the patient should be made, to discover injuries caused by the initial fall; wounds of the scalp and even fractures are not uncommon complications of a fit.

Encouragement and rest. The natural tendency for sleep should be encouraged, but the first aider must arrange for the patient to be watched in case the fit recurs.

Promoting comfort. If temporary removal to a suitable shelter is possible – as, for example, to a neighbouring house – the patient should be made comfortable in bed with extra wraps, and the room kept quiet and darkened. A non-stimulating drink, such as diluted milk, may be given (providing no injury has been sustained). The patient should be kept under close observation for several hours, as behaviour during recovery may be abnormal.

Medical aid. The services of a doctor should be obtained immediately if the patient shows a tendency to recurring fits; in any case, the first aider should advise his patient to obtain medical treatment.

Minor epilepsy or petit mal

This is a less serious form of the disease, in which a patient is seized with an attack of unconsciousness but there are no convulsions. Suddenly, perhaps in the course of a conversation, the patient will stop speaking and his eyes will appear to have become fixed, with a dreamy stare.

The attack may be so slight as not to be noticed, except by a careful observer and the patient himself. The disease is of importance, for it may develop into major epilepsy, or an attack may be followed by any of the complications of the major disease. No treatment other than medical attendance is required.

Post-epileptic complications

Automatism

Occasionally after an epileptic fit, instead of the normal return to consciousness, the patient may perform an action of which he is entirely ignorant at the time and which he cannot recall afterwards: e.g. he may commence undressing, or even act violently towards bystanders.

Mania

Temporary insanity may occasionally follow a fit. The first aider will appreciate that his primary duty when confronted by a post-epileptic complication is to restrain the patient from doing harm to himself or others, pending the arrival of medical aid.

STROKE

Stroke is the common term for a condition of altered consciousness occurring suddenly, usually in elderly people, due to haemorrhage into the substance of the brain (cerebral haemorrhage) or clotting of one of the brain's blood vessels (cerebral thrombosis).

Causes

This condition may be associated with high blood pressure or hardening of the arteries. Patients susceptible to a stroke may experience warning symptoms for some time prior to the onset of the seizure. Giddiness, persistent headaches, shortness of breath, and nose-bleeding should call attention to the possibility of raised blood pressure. If medical attention is sought at this stage, strokes may be prevented by treating the high blood pressure with suitable drugs.

Symptoms and signs

A stroke may occur at night, when the patient is resting or asleep, or after exertion. The patient may be seized by sudden headache or giddiness or may collapse without warning. He may develop complete or partial loss of consciousness, or simply become confused or disorientated.

The temperature of the body is raised and the face may be flushed. The pulse is usually slow and strong, and the breathing becomes characteristic, being accompanied by snores and puffing out of the cheeks on expiration.

The pupils may become unequal and fail to respond to light, while the head and eyes are often turned towards the affected side of the brain.

It is well known that a stroke is usually followed by paralysis of one side of the body and, even in the stage of unconsciousness, the affected side will often be found to be more limp than its opposite, while the corresponding cheek is smooth and puffed out. Incontinence of urine and convulsions may occasionally occur. It should be noted that the symptoms and signs of stroke are very similiar to those that occur in compression of the brain.

Diagnosis

It may be stated that stroke is the commonest cause of insensibility in patients over the age of forty-five, and since first aid diagnosis is only intended to be provisional in character, little harm will be done to an elderly patient who is found unconscious by assuming that he is suffering from a stroke and treating for this condition before medical aid arrives.

It is important to exclude the possibility of poisoning or diabetes, but this is usually easy, for in these cases clues suggesting poisoning are often found, while the circumstances in which the patient is taken ill (for example, while obviously on his way to work) generally point to the onset of a sudden illness rather than an attempted suicide.

Confusion of stroke with the state of alcoholism, however, has frequently occurred in practice, and it must be emphasized that the mere smell of alcohol on the breath does not in itself merit a diagnosis of drunkenness, for a patient may have been feeling ill at the onset of the fit and purposely taken an alcoholic drink.

The first aider must not be misled by a rapid return to consciousness, for in a number of cases there is a quick recovery, but the patient remains extremely susceptible to recurrence.

It must also be remembered that not every case of stroke conforms to the type described above, and various modifications are possible according to the area of the brain affected. Thus, sudden loss of speech occurs in certain forms of stroke, although there may be no other paralysis.

Treatment

The golden rule in the treatment of a case of suspected stroke is to examine the patient as little as possible and to avoid moving him more than is absolutely necessary. Thus, wherever possible, the patient should be allowed to remain lying where he has fallen. It is quite feasible, for example, in the home, to make up a bed on the floor and carefully to move the patient on to it. Any attempt to carry the patient upstairs may easily end fatally by increasing the haemorrhage.

If it is essential to move a patient, as when the seizure has occurred in the street, careful and gentle handling is essential if bleeding is to be kept to its minimum.

Airway. Maintenance of the patient's airway is as always of prime importance. The recovery position should be used for the unconscious patient.

Care of the mouth. False teeth should be removed and carefully preserved. If the mouth is allowed to fill up with saliva there is always the risk that some of the saliva may be sucked down into the lungs and cause bronchopneumonia, a common and often fatal complication.

Warmth. The patient should be covered with a blanket, and suitable wraps placed under him and tucked well in at the sides and feet. Care should be taken not to allow the patient to lie on keys, coins, or other sharp objects.

Masterly inactivity is the most important treatment to adopt after the above procedures have been undertaken. It comprises doing absolutely nothing beyond watching the patient and appreciating the fact that additional treatments, such as trying to give stimulants or medicine, will do more harm than good. Masterly inactivity is one of the most difficult treatments to apply in medical work and first aid.

Medical advice is always essential, since some cases in younger people are treated at certain special hospitals by a surgical operation on the blood vessels in or around the brain.

INFANTILE CONVULSIONS

Fits occurring in infants and children are known as infantile convulsions. The complaint is most common up to the age of eighteen months, but convulsions may occur in older children.

Causes

The most common cause precipitating a convulsion in the pre-school child is a sudden fever, the nature of the infection being less important than the speed and height of the temperature.

There are other potential causes, such as hypoglycaemia, meningitis, tetany, intracranial haemorrhage, ear infection, reaction to drugs, and teething.

Symptoms

An infant liable to develop a fit will often show signs of general nervous irritability for some time before the actual onset of convulsions. Thus it may be somewhat jerky in its manner, and restless. The actual signs of the fit itself may be summarized as follows:

Breath-holding. The infant develops irregularity in breathing, or may stop breathing for a second or two.

Rigidity. He throws his head back and becomes stiff all over.

Altered colour. Alteration in the colour of the face may vary, from slight pallor or sallowness to marked blueness of the face or limbs.

Twitching. The infant may not exhibit true convulsions as have been described in epilepsy. Some twitching of the body will, however, be noticed in the majority of cases.

Squinting and frothing at the mouth are occasional signs.

Treatment

It must be remembered that fits in childhood cause alarm to parents but are only rarely fatal. The parents should be reassured, therefore, that the child will soon recover and that there is no need for them to worry whilst medical aid is being sought.

General measures to protect the convulsive child from harming himself are most important. Where there is high fever, tepid sponging or fanning may bring down the temperature and prevent further fitting.

Send for medical aid to determine the cause of the fit and obtain advice as to aftercare.

FAINTING (SYNCOPE)

Fainting or syncope is a state of temporary unconsciousness due to diminished blood supply to the brain. The cerebral ischaemia may be due to any of the following causes, which are frequently combined:
1. Exhaustion, lack of food, or exertion while in a state of fatigue.
2. Emotion, especially fright or fear.
3. Accidents, including minor accidents, especially those involving loss of blood.
4. Lack of fresh air; close atmosphere and heat.
5. Posture, e.g. standing for a long time on a hot day or suddenly standing upright after resting.

Symptoms and signs

The patient feels giddy, swoons and falls to the ground. The face is pale, the skin cold, clammy and covered with sweat. The pulse is quick and feeble and may become almost imperceptible at the wrist.

Treatment

Lay the patient down. A quick examination must be made to exclude the presence of haemorrhage, e.g. burst varicose veins. Any bleeding must be arrested before treating the faint. In the absence of haemorrhage the treatment is as follows:

Position. The patient should be kept lying down with his head and shoulders low, and the feet raised and supported in an elevated position. If unable to lie down, the head may be placed down between the knees, but recovery is quicker when the patient is lying flat.

Warmth. Covering the patient with blankets or with coats, etc., borrowed from bystanders will prevent him becoming cold or wet, should this be a problem.

Clothing. Tight clothing round the neck, chest and waist must be loosened or removed.

Space. Instruct bystanders to avoid crowding the patient. If it is necessary to remove the patient from a crowded room, a stretcher should be used.

Fluids. On return to consciousness, hot tea or coffee, to which sugar has been added, may be given in sips, but it is undesirable to give too much at a time owing to the risk of vomiting.

DIABETES MELLITUS

Diabetic patients are always liable to lose consciousness due to a progressively decreasing amount of sugar in the blood (hypoglycaemia). The effect of low blood sugar may be quite rapid, and circumstances in which it has not been possible to obtain adequate food, due perhaps to a long journey or delays, are very liable to precipitate an attack.

On the other hand, though this is much rarer, patients may over-inject themselves with insulin or fail to take the meal which should follow within half an hour of the injection. This results in the same effect, also due to low blood sugar. Patients on oral anti-diabetic drugs may also suffer hypoglycaemia if a meal is missed.

Hypoglycaemic coma (low blood sugar)

Diagnosis

There may be a history of missing or irregular meals, unaccustomed exercise or an overdose of insulin. Behaviour before may be quite normal, or may resemble or be mistaken for drunkenness.

The face is pale and the skin shows profuse sweating when blood sugar is very low. Breathing is shallow and the pulse rapid, though this may become weaker and difficult to feel as unconsciousness approaches.

Treatment

Provided the patient is still conscious and can swallow, the treatment is simple and recovery dramatic. The ability to swallow can be tested by tipping a spoonful of water into the side of the mouth. If this is swallowed, he should be given a heaped dessertspoonful of sugar in half a cup of water. This should be repeated if recovery is not complete.

The patient must lie down and rest quietly.

If the patient is already unconscious a doctor may give the sugar solution via the rectum or intravenously. Nothing should be given by mouth.

Most diabetics carry sugar with them in anticipation of an impending hypoglycaemic attack.

Hypoglycaemic coma may occur quite rapidly. Once the patient is unconscious, fits may occur, and urgent medical help is required to prevent serious brain damage.

Rebound low blood sugar is possible, so the patient should be checked by a doctor.

Hyperglycaemic coma (high blood sugar)

This very much rarer emergency may result from lack of insulin. It is usually precipitated by illness, excitement, fatigue or over-indulgence. It is much less likely to occur without warning, and is usually preceded by a variable period of ill health.

Diagnosis

The skin is dry and the patient complains of headache and increasing drowsiness, which deepens into coma. Breathing becomes prolonged and sighing with 'air hunger'. The breathing has a characteristic smell of nail varnish (acetone) and reflexes are diminished. The patient's tongue is very dry and he may complain of thirst.

Treatment

Medical aid should be sought as quickly as possible, or the patient urgently removed to hospital. Meanwhile, he should be kept warm and quiet. If there is doubt about cause of decreased conscious level in a known diabetic, the administration of a sugary drink to the patient (providing he can take it) is safer whilst awaiting medical help: this will do no harm and may help, as confusion may easily occur between hyper- and hypoglycaemia.

URAEMIA

Uraemia is the term applied to a serious complication of kidney disease, due to an accumulation of poisonous substances in the bloodstream which would normally be removed from the body by the kidneys. Uraemia may take several forms, e.g.:
1. Increasing drowsiness leading to a deep sleep; this is by far the commonest form.
2. Recurrent fits occurring in elderly people are suggestive of this complication.
3. A seizure resembling stroke.
4. Coma, with distressed respiration.
Patients suffering from uraemia are usually already under medical care, which has been sought as a result of warning symptoms. It is necessary, therefore, to summon medical aid immediately, and in the meantime to keep the patient quiet, warm and comfortable.

Coma due to uraemia is very unlikely in a previously healthy patient.

UNCONSCIOUSNESS AS AN EFFECT OF TEMPERATURE (see also Chapter 27)

Heat stroke
Heat exhaustion
Hypothermia

—27

The Effects of Temperature

Extremes of heat or cold can cause severe damage to skin and the underlying tissues. The body's ability to control the 'core' temperature may be lost and unconsciousness may occur. (The control of body temperature is reviewed in Chapter 14.)

THE EFFECTS OF COLD

The body will attempt to maintain the core temperature by reducing blood flow to the skin. In extreme cold, or following immersion in cold water, this defence mechanism is lost. Shivering occurs early, but this rapidly becomes ineffective at extremes of cold.

The effects can be subdivided as follows:
1. Local effects, e.g. frostbite.
2. General effects, e.g. hypothermia.

Local effects

Most frequently affected are the nose, ears, hands and feet. Superficial damage may occur in a few seconds in extreme cold. If deeper tissues under the skin are frozen, the cells may die and the blood supply may be permanently affected with the development of gangrene.

Symptoms and signs

1. Increasing pain with numbness.
2. Inability to move or control the part.
3. The skin becomes blotchy or waxy white.

Treatment

1. Remove the casualty to shelter; lay him down as soon as possible. **Gradual** rewarming is essential to prevent further damage. The casualty will not be able to feel trauma to the affected part. He may rub or squeeze it in an attempt to obtain sensation. This should be prevented if possible and the casualty not allowed to walk on cold-injured feet unless this may endanger the survival of other members of the party.

2. Remove clothing **gently. Do not rub affected parts.** Remove rings, watches etc. if possible.

3. Warm affected hands by placing them in the casualty's own armpits. Affected feet may be warmed by contact with the rescuer's skin. Facial areas should be warmed by skin contact also. Cover with a warm anorak to prevent heat loss.

4. **Tepid** water may be used if available. It must not be too hot (it should be tested like a baby's feeding bottle).

Radiant heat, e.g. electric fires, must not be used.

5. **Elevate** affected limbs.

6. Seek medical aid as soon as possible.

General effects

Body temperature

1. Normal temperature = 37°C ± 1 degree.
2. Moderate hypothermia = 30–35°C.
3. Profound hypothermia = <30°C.

Hypothermia is likely to be irreversible below 25°C. It should be noted that a clinical thermometer capable of sub-normal readings is required to measure temperatures below 35°C.

Wetting reduces the insulation value of the casualty's clothing to almost nothing. Heat loss is rapidly increased by exposure to windy conditions, especially when clothing and skin are wet. Alcohol may also increase heat loss.

Symptoms and signs

Early:
1. Feeling of intense cold.
2. Pallor and/or cyanosis of the extremities.
3. Shivering, which becomes uncontrollable.

Later:
4. Shivering is replaced by the inability to move limbs properly, and slurred speech with dulling of mental faculties. **The casualty may not realize he is in danger.**
5. Disorientation.
6. Slow pulse and respiration rate.
7. Complete unconsciousness, absent pulse and respiration.
8. Pupils may be dilated.

The casualty may appear dead. Any person *apparently* **dead who could be hypothermic must be given resuscitation until medical help arrives.**

Treatment

1. Place in the recovery position (place infants on their sides).
2. Cover with insulating material such as anoraks and blankets.
3. Remove wet clothes if possible. Dry clothes will retain heat much better. Place the casualty in a sleeping bag, polythene rescue bag or Flectalon® rescue blanket, as available. Foil blankets have a place provided all wet clothing has been removed. Large plastic bags such as dustbin liners can prevent wind chill. Cover the patient up to the neck with the plastic bags and ensure that the head (but **not** the face) is covered with insulating material, especially in babies.
4. Arrange removal from the cold environment, especially if at high altitude.
5. If consciousness improves and the casualty is rational, warm drinks may be given.
6. **Warm** water bottles (not hot) may be applied to the trunk but not the limbs, since this may cause blood to be diverted away from vital organs. If no medical help is likely for some hours and the facility is available, place the **trunk**, but not the limbs, in a bath of water at 40°C. This temperature should be maintained by stirring in additional warm water from time to time.

Immersion in warm water may be dangerous and should not be attempted unless medical help is not expected to arrive for several hours.
Do not administer alcohol.

7. If there is no pulse or detectable respiration commence cardiopulmonary resuscitation.

The extremes of age

Hypothermia occurs readily at the extremes of age, when the body's defence mechanisms against cold function less well. The elderly often take inadequate quantities of food or warm drinks and may not be able to afford fuel to heat their homes adequately. Hypothermic infants may look deceptively well but may appear lethargic and refuse to feed. **These may be the only signs of hypothermia in a baby.**

THE EFFECTS OF HEAT

The body's defences against excess heating are:
1. Increasing blood flow to the skin.
2. Increasing sweat production.
3. Increasing the respiratory rate.
The latter two cause increased evaporation of water resulting in a cooling effect. The effects of overheating may be mild or severe:

1. Mild, e.g. heat exhaustion.
2. Severe, e.g. heat stroke.

Heat exhaustion

This is due to depletion of salt and water. It primarily affects those unused to hot environments and may be precipitated by an attack of diarrhoea and vomiting (traveller's diarrhoea). Heat exhaustion can occur in marathons and fun runs, even in temperate climates.

Symptoms and signs

1. The patient feels exhausted and faint.
2. There may be dizziness and nausea.
3. Moist, 'clammy' skin.
4. Rapid pulse, becoming weaker.
5. Rapid respiration.
6. The body temperature is usually not much raised.

Treatment

1. Prevent the casualty from moving about; lay him down in a cool place.
2. If fainting has not occurred, allow sips of water containing half a teaspoon of common (table) salt and one of sugar to each pint (approximately half a litre) of water. Proprietary sachets are now available.
3. Maintain the casualty semi-recumbent or lying down until recovery occurs.

Heat stroke

The condition follows exposure to high environmental temperatures and humidity or severe fever. It occurs when the 'core' body temperature rises and the defence mechanisms become inadequate. Humid conditions reduce the evaporation of sweat and aggravate the condition.

Symptoms and signs

1. The victim feels hot, restless and may complain of headache.
2. There may be sudden loss of consciousness.
3. Usually the skin is warm and rather dry; the patient appears flushed.
4. The heart rate is rapid with a strong pulse.
5. The 'core' temperature is high and may reach 40°C or more.

Treatment

1. Do not allow the casualty to move. Make him lie down in a cool environment.
2. Wet the casualty all over with cold, but not iced, water. This is facilitated by wrapping him in a sheet. Keep the sheet wet to increase heat loss.
3. Fan the casualty's face but **not** the whole body, as rapid cooling will cause constriction of blood vessels in the skin and may actually reduce heat loss.
4. Summon urgent medical assistance.
5. If the casualty is unconscious, place him in the recovery position.
6. It is unwise to allow the casualty to drink until the temperature falls to 38°C or less, as sudden loss of consciousness may result in regurgitation and inhalation of gastric contents.

— 28

Poisons

A poison is any substance which is liable to have a harmful effect on the human body, injuring health or destroying life.

A poison may enter the body through the mouth, by inhalation, through the skin or by injection. The poisoning may be accidental, intentional or homicidal. In practice, as well as finding an ill person, there may be evidence of poisoning by the presence of suspicious bottles, pills or a suicide note. If suicide or homicide is in any way suspected, care should be taken not to remove or destroy any likely evidence, though the welfare of the victim must be the foremost consideration.

Parasuicide

Another common type of self-poisoning is termed parasuicide. A young person who is emotionally disturbed may take what they believe to be a less than fatal amount of a poison, such as a painkiller or sleeping tablet, in such a manner that others are immediately aware of what has been done. The object is to obtain attention and to try and solve the emotional problem, rather than to take their life.

Recovery is the rule, but care should be taken to give the necessary first aid and to obtain medical advice as soon as possible.

Fatal poisoning

In recent years the pattern of poisoning has changed, and today the incidence of fatal poisoning in Britain is roughly:

$$
75\% \left\{ \begin{array}{l} \text{sleeping tablets} \\ \text{aspirin} \\ \text{paracetamol} \\ \text{other painkillers} \\ \text{antidepressants} \\ \text{carbon monoxide} \end{array} \right.
$$

25% other

The causes of fatal poisoning vary widely in different countries, depending on the substances available.

As far as first aid treatment for serious poisoning is concerned, it is important to distinguish between those poisons which are corrosive and burn the mouth, and those which are not. The difference is usually obvious.

First aid treatment in poisoning

The immediate requirement is to ensure that respiration and circulation are maintained. If resuscitation is required, the presence of any poison on the face, or which is likely to be in the exhaled breath, might indicate the need for a manual method or special protection, e.g. Brook airway (see Chapter 5) or gauze coverings, if the exhaled air method is used.

The next requirement is to determine what type of poison has been used and act as follows:

1. If the poison is a corrosive which will cause burning of the lips, mouth or tongue, or is a paraffin or a petroleum product (which though fairly harmless in the stomach would cause grave damage inhaled with vomit), then do not make the patient vomit but send quickly to hospital.

2. The unconscious patient should not be given anything by mouth, and should not be made to vomit. The patient should be placed in the recovery position as soon as a clear airway has been established and the patient has a satisfactory pulse and respiration. If these are not satisfactory, the patient will have to be resuscitated.

3. With all other poisons, the conscious patient can be made to vomit by passing a finger down the victim's throat, provided the patient is not uncooperative. This should be done with the patient leaning so far forward that the head is below the chest. Do not persevere with this if it does not produce a result.

The above general rules apply particularly when the specific poison is not known. If the poison is known, it may be possible to modify the treatment to good effect. The use of specific antidotes in first aid is limited. The general commonsense measures which are applicable in all first aid work are usually sufficient to preserve life and cope with the immediate emergency in cases of poisoning.

COMMON POISONS

Sleeping tablets

Tablets given to relieve anxiety or promote sleep (benzodiazepines, e.g. Valium, and in some cases barbiturates) can be taken in intentional overdose by adults, and may be taken accidentally by children.

The patient sinks into sleep which may deepen into coma, with respiratory depression, low blood pressure, a quick and feeble pulse and cold skin.

Treatment

The unconscious patient should be placed in the recovery position. Early admission to hospital should be arranged, but meanwhile the first aider should be on the look-out for respiratory failure and be prepared to give artificial respiration and oxygen if available.

Paracetamol

This painkilling drug can cause severe and possibly fatal liver damage if taken in overdose. The patient may vomit, but does not lapse into coma and may feel perfectly well for over 24 hours.

Treatment

Medical treatment can prevent the liver damage but must be given within twelve hours to be effective. The patient must be urgently brought under medical care – even if there are no symptoms – so that blood paracetamol can be measured and treatment given if necessary.

Aspirin

Aspirin is sometimes used in large doses for a suicidal attempt. It may produce vomiting which lessens absorption, but can affect the central nervous system, producing confusion, over-breathing, sweating, ringing in the ears and sometimes deafness. Coma is rare. There may be abdominal pains, and extensive gastric bleeding may also occur.

Treatment

Because of the slow rate of absorption, an emetic is often effective, and a doctor may wash out the stomach with good results. If a large dose has been taken, or there has been marked absorption of the drug, specialist hospital treatment is essential.

Antidepressants

These drugs are prescribed for the relief of depression, and a suicidally depressed patient may take them in overdose. The patient may initially be excitable but will usually lapse into a deep coma. Depressed respiration, a fast heart rate and convulsions are possible.

Treatment

Help should be sought urgently, as death can occur. The patient should be kept in the recovery position.

Carbon monoxide

The circumstances usually point to this form of poisoning. Common sources are exhaust fumes from petrol engines, and fumes from solid fuel or gas fires. It may be accidental or suicidal.

The patient experiences giddiness, headache and tightness of the chest followed by vomiting, collapse and unconsciousness. When found, the victim often has a characteristic pink appearance and may have stopped breathing.

Treatment

The deeply unconscious patient should be dragged out into the fresh air and given exhaled air resuscitation. Pure oxygen should be given as soon as it can be made available.

OTHER POISONS

Narcotics (heroin, morphine and other compounds related to opium)

These are valuable drugs for the treatment of pain and other disorders, but can be taken in overdose or abused, and may lead to addiction. Overdose will produce drowsiness, gradually passing into coma. The patient will have pinpoint pupils, and respiratory depression – in this case a slowing or irregularity of respiration – may occur. Treatment is urgent in severe cases, and resuscitation should be commenced. Trained personnel may give naloxone 0.4 to 1.2 mg intravenously to an adult or $10 \mu g$ $(0.01 \, mg)$ per kilogram to children. This is an antidote which produces a rapid reversal of poisoning. Medical advice should be sought urgently, and the patient should be kept under observation.

Solvents

Volatile substances which give off a vapour (e.g. petrol, waxes, glues and solvents) may be swallowed or inhaled. If swallowed, the patient should not be made to vomit, as these substances may be very harmful if even a small amount is accidentally inhaled into the lungs.

Solvent abuse

Volatile substances may be abused by being inhaled for 'pleasure'. This practice, often called glue sniffing, may lead to drowsiness, hallucinations, vomiting, convulsions, coma and cardiac arrest, though in most cases it has no serious adverse effects. A young person may be found collapsed after an episode of sniffing. The first aider should decide if resuscitation is necessary. If the patient is breathing and has a good pulse, he should be placed in the recovery position and help should be sought.

Treatment

If the substance has been swallowed, on no account must the patient be made to vomit. He should be given nothing by mouth and should rest quietly awaiting medical advice. If it has been inhaled, hospital care is particularly essential to preserve the lungs and maintain oxygenation.

Insecticides

Poisoning from insecticides often results from careless usage. It may follow accidental inhalation after spillage on the skin. In such cases, contaminated clothing should be removed and the skin washed with soap and water.

On inhalation, the organophosphate insecticides cause excess salivation and sweating, difficulty in breathing, constricted pupils and a slow pulse. Artificial respiration may be needed and the specific antidote is intramuscular injection of 2 mg atropine sulphate. This may be found in the first aid kit where such chemicals are used and may be given by the first aider as a life saving measure and repeated if necessary.

Corrosives

These may be acid or alkaline, and if swallowed produce a burning pain in the mouth, throat, neck, chest and abdomen. The portions of skin and mucous membrane which are affected are inflamed, and may be stained. There may be bloodstained vomit and, later, diarrhoea. The patient becomes profoundly ill and may have difficulty in speaking or breathing.

Treatment

Three to four cups of water or milk should be given by mouth at once. Emetics should not be given, not only because the vomit may cause further burning, but because of the danger of perforating the stomach or oesophagus. Once in hospital, which must be reached as quickly as possible, the stomach may be washed out and treatment given for pain and other complications.

Food poisoning

Eating food which has putrefied or which has been contaminated by a chemical is a common cause of poisoning.

Symptoms and signs such as pain, vomiting and later diarrhoea appear after taking the meal, and may simultaneously affect several patients who have eaten the same food. A patient suffering from food poisoning may have noticed an unusual taste in the food which he took.

Treatment

The patient should be seen by a doctor, as the young and elderly can get very ill very quickly from vomiting and diarrhoea.

Berries and fungi

Children are occasionally affected through eating poisonous berries, e.g. those of the deadly nightshade, or toadstools taken by mistake for mushrooms. In these cases, symptoms of poisoning often occur soon after the food has been eaten.

In children, staining of the mouth and, possibly, the clothing may supply evidence that poisonous berries have been eaten.

Treatment

The patient should be taken to the hospital. A specimen of the berries or fungi should also be taken if posssible.

Alcohol

Alcohol is often thought of as a stimulant, but in fact it depresses the nervous system. Someone who is drunk may be aggressive, with slurred speech and poor coordination, and is at risk of injury through loss of control. Many fatal road traffic accidents are caused by the effects of alcohol on drivers and pedestrians.

Note: any person found unconscious and with breath smelling of alcohol may not be suffering from alcohol excess but from a head injury, and should be carefully examined for external signs of injury.

Recovery from moderate alcohol intoxication takes a few hours, and if the patient is conscious, the main first aid measure is to prevent the patient injuring himself or interfering with others. Larger amounts of alcohol are capable of causing a deep coma, which can be fatal. The skin may be flushed and the pulse weak. The body is very relaxed. The tongue can fall back and block the airway, and vomit may also obstruct the airway. It is therefore most important to keep the severely intoxicated patient in the recovery position, and to seek medical advice.

Industrial poisoning

Certain chemicals employed in industry are liable to produce harmful effects. The substances concerned may cause a skin irritation (dermatitis), or may enter the body and then produce general symptoms and signs of poisoning. Most factories now employ Medical Officers or State Registered Nurses who undertake overriding responsibility for the welfare of the workers, and who give such instructions as they think fit to first aid personnel.

Industrial chemicals which enter the body usually gain access through the respiratory system; fumes or a dust may be inhaled. Sometimes, however, absorption occurs through the mouth and digestive system; this may result from carelessness, e.g. when an employee who is working with a poisonous chemical fails to take personal precautions such as washing his hands before eating.

Many cases of industrial poisoning result from the repeated absorption of small doses of a chemical which accumulates within the body. For this reason, symptoms and signs usually develop gradually, and may differ considerably from those which are caused by the administration of a single large dose (such as occurs in the accidental and suicidal cases). When fumes, including gases and vapours, are inhaled, however, sudden and severe symptoms may develop.

The harmful chemicals commonly used in factories may be briefly classified as follows:

1. **Inorganic (simple) chemicals**, e.g. lead, arsenic, phosphorus, mercury, chromic acid and radioactive substances.
2. **Organic (complicated) chemicals**, e.g. aniline, trinitrotoluene, asbestos, etc.
3. **Poisonous gases**:
    (a) asphyxiants, e.g. carbon monoxide, carbon dioxide;
    (b) irritants, e.g. nitrous fumes, ammonia, etc.;
    (c) toxic vapours given off from volatile solvents.

Prevention of industrial poisoning

In most countries, there is an organization under government direction which is constantly engaged in safeguarding the health of those who work in factories where harmful substances are used.

Regulations are in force which ensure that the best possible means of protection are provided for the workers to prevent cases of poisoning. Suitable measures include efficient ventilation of workshops, supplying special respirators for the use of employees, and avoiding as far as possible methods of work which create dust which might be inhaled.

In addition, the employees of certain factories (where particularly toxic chemicals are used) are examined at regular intervals by the appointed factory doctor, so that the first signs of ill health can be detected and prompt measures undertaken to prevent actual poisoning.

Sometimes a first aider who works in a factory may be asked to inspect the workers regularly, during the intervals between the doctor's visits. This is a most important duty. The first aider must familiarize himself with the first symptoms and signs which may indicate exposure to the substances in use, and must promptly refer to the doctor any suspicious case which he may discover.

A valuable method of preventing industrial poisoning is to educate employees so that they understand the dangers to which they are exposed, and are aware of the best means of personal protection.

Childhood poisoning

Small children are naturally inquisitive, and often put the things they find into their mouths. When the substance is a medicine, a household chemical or a plant leaf or berry, poisoning may occur. This kind of poisoning is called 'accidental' because it is unintentional, though unfortunately non-accidental poisoning can also occur (when a parent or guardian intentionally poisons a child). The peak age for accidental poisoning is two years, though it can occur from just under one year to four years of age. Prevention is very important. Tablets, alcohol and household and garden chemicals should not be left lying within reach.

Antidepressants, tablets for diarrhoea, aspirin and iron tablets cause the most serious poisoning, and even the taking of one or two tablets could be dangerous. Most cases involve some doubt as to whether anything has even been taken, but every case should be taken seriously even though there may be no symptoms. If the child is conscious it should be made to vomit by inserting a finger in its throat, after first putting it over the first aider's knee with its head lower than its seat. The vomit should be kept for inspection, and an opinion should be obtained on the likely seriousness of the case; in many cases the substance taken is not poisonous at all.

29

Psychogenic Ailments

The mind is liable to many disorders, some of which are of interest and importance to the first aider. They fall loosely into two groups, neuroses and psychoses.

Neurosis

There are many kinds of neurosis, just as there are many varieties of illness. Some neuroses are mild and comprise symptoms such as insomnia, nightmares, general irritability, depression and unnecessary anxiety; more severe cases include the anxiety states and certain forms of hysteria.

The characteristic feature of most neuroses is that the patient realizes that his nerves are bad, and for this reason applies to a doctor for treatment.

Psychosis

This is a mental disorder which is popularly known as derangement of the mind. The characteristic feature is that the patient fails to appreciate the realities of life, and does not realize that he is ill and requires treatment.

In many psychoses, the patient develops false ideas or beliefs. These are called delusions. Other patients develop hallucinations, i.e. they see imaginary people or animals, or hear voices.

It should be noted that many neuroses and psychoses can be cured by skilled psychiatric treatment.

Normal instincts

It is well known that the human body is endowed with a number of feelings which are designed to protect life; if hungry man will take food, if in pain he will take avoiding action. Similar senses exist in the mind; of these, one of the most important is that of fear.

Fear

This is a natural emotion, ensuring an attempt to avoid danger either by flight or concealment.

A baby begins its life with the ability to fear, but it has to learn when and for what reasons to become afraid. While the right kind of fear is valuable because it is designed to protect life, it is unfortunately only too easy for unnecessary and irrational fears to be imparted to children. For example, a mother terrified of thunderstorms creates a similar fear in her offspring.

The symptoms and signs of fear are well known, and include an anxious expression, a change in colour of the face, dryness of the mouth, sweating, rapid breathing and palpitations. There may be irritability, trembling (tremors), and in some people looseness of the bowels. These symptoms are often accompanied by a desire to run away and seek safety from the danger. With experience, the normal human being learns how to deal with fear.

Generally the effects of fear are transient, and soon disappear when the emergency has ceased; even if danger remains or is repeated, most people quickly return to their normal state, especially when engaged in useful and important work.

The duty of a first aider when dealing with a case of fear or terror is quite clear. He must provide, as far as possible, security from the danger, and adopt a sympathetic attitude towards the patient, explaining that fear is only natural and will soon pass off.

Anxiety states

An anxiety state is a neurosis which is characterized by the symptoms and signs of fear out of all proportion to the factors precipitating them. The patient may or may not be able to identify precipitating factors accurately.

Mild anxiety states are common in civil life, and many persons troubled in this way obtain successful results from medical treatment. Milder cases may not realize that they are suffering from anything more serious than 'nerves'. For these reasons, the anxiety states which occur in normal civil life do not come within the scope of first aid.

Under stress and strain, however, patients suffering from anxiety may become worse and are liable to develop attacks of terror, called panic. A patient who is suffering from an anxiety state, even a mild one, is also liable to become accident prone.

Confusional states

These, as the name implies, are mental conditions in which a patient becomes confused in his manner, behaviour, or ideas. The patient will be disorientated in time, place, or person to some extent.

Mild confusion is common in the delirium which accompanies a severe illness, e.g. pneumonia. That which follows concussion or an epileptic fit may be more severe; these examples, however, are not usually included under the definition. Other causes are drugs, alcohol, brain tumours and toxic states.

In a true confusional state the patient looks bewildered; he is unable to think clearly or to understand what is said to him. His memory is usually muddled and he may be unable to recall his name and address, or such simple facts as the time of the year, the job in which he is employed, etc. A person more severely affected may suffer from hallucinations; that is, he may think that he hears a voice speaking to him. Sometimes fear is a prominent symptom, and in this event the patient may become restless or even violent.

Mental symptoms are often accompanied by signs of general ill health, e.g. fever, a 'dirty' tongue, and an unhealthy appearance. Such patients should be reassured and protected from self-harm, and medical help should be sought.

Hysteria

This is a neurosis which may show itself in several forms:
1. Hysterical conversion, which may include such manipulations as loss of voice, or paralysis or loss of sensation in a limb.
2. Loss of memory.
3. Unconsciousness without signs of illness or injury.

It must be stressed that in true hysteria, the condition is very real to the patient even though no physical cause can be found.

Hysterical fits

These are very uncommon in practice, but are liable to occur in a susceptible subject as a result of a sudden emotional strain, e.g. fear.

The patient falls suddenly to the ground and may lose all consciousness of his surroundings. He may writhe on the floor, laugh or scream continuously and resist help by struggling. After a variable length of time he suddenly or gradually recovers consciousness, or else passes into a deep sleep. Usually he has no recollection afterwards of what he has been doing or thinking during the attack.

At the first sign of a fit, the patient should be firmly treated. Sympathy should be avoided. If the fit continues he should be moved to a new environment under the care of a skilled attendant. It is often very difficult to differentiate between true and hysterical fits. In **both** cases the prime objective is to prevent harm coming to the patient.

First aid treatment of psychogenic illness

1. Remove the patient to a place where he feels safe, away from people and bustle.

2. Reassure convincingly.
3. Keep under continuous observation.
4. Make sure there is no physical injury. A patient in this state will not be able to tell the first aider if he is hurt.
5. Give non-stimulating drinks, i.e. avoid coffee and alcohol.
6. Obtain medical help as soon as possible.

Depression

The term depression covers a whole spectrum of psychological disturbances, ranging from common, mild depression (a reaction to life events, experienced by many normal people at some time) to the very profound state of withdrawal which characterizes the serious psychotic depressive illness. In its severe forms this may be accompanied by apathy, loss of interest in life, work, hobbies or family, feelings of guilt or self-hate. The patient may even suffer delusions about himself or others or his surroundings. There may be total withdrawal from reality. All this may be accompanied by anxiety. There may also be associated physical symptoms, such as loss of appetite, weight loss, constipation, disturbed sleep (especially early morning wakening) and loss of libido. All this may be totally out of proportion to, or devoid of, precipitating causes.

The patient's speech may be slow and his appearance unkempt. He may appear openly unhappy and tearful, or simply detached and uncommunicative. Some patients display very little in the way of depression to the outside world, but in all cases feelings of hopelessness for the future may lead to suicidal ideas and a real danger of self-harm or suicide.

Treatment can be very successful and ranges from simple discussion and support to antidepressant therapy or ECT (electroconvulsive therapy). Severe cases may require admission to hospital for treatment or close observation, especially when there is a high suicidal risk.

The very nature of a severe depressive illness often means that the patient does not have the drive to seek medical help for himself, and must be encouraged to do so. In severe cases it may be necessary to detain a patient in hospital against his wishes, until treatment enables the dangerous suicidal period to pass. The law allows this via the Mental Health Act, which enables doctors, relatives and social workers to admit and treat a patient who is in such a severe pathological state of depression that he is unable to seek such help voluntarily. These cases are fortunately rare.

30

Burns

Burn wounds are a common cause of pain, disability and disfigurement, but they can often be prevented by attention to detail, e.g. when dealing with open fires and loose dresses, boiling water and hot tea or coffee. Legislation to ban flammable nightdresses led to a large decrease in the number of girls injured by a burning nightdress, but cotton dresses are just as dangerous. Care when using open petrol and paraffin stoves is vital. Good accident prevention is an essential part of first aid training.

The burn wound

This is caused through damage to the skin by heat, chemicals or radiation. A burn is caused by dry heat and a scald by wet heat, but there is no fundamental difference in the nature of the damage. The single expression 'burn' will include all. The damage to the skin involves all layers of the skin, but particularly the growing epithelial element. Damage to the capillaries causes them to ooze serum, and a large quantity of body fluids escapes through the skin surface, and into the depth of the skin.

There are two main factors to be considered in burns: depth, and per cent of body surface burnt.

Burns are classified according to their depth (Fig. 30.1):

1. **Erythema** is a reddening of the skin, for example as seen in sunburn.
2. **Partial skin loss** involves the epidermis and part of the dermis. Blisters are formed; the surface looks pink and is painful, but if kept sterile it will heal spontaneously.
3. **Whole skin loss** involves the full depth of the dermis, including the hair follicles and sweat glands. The burn is white, dead and insensitive and will heal from the edges only.

The depth of burn depends on the temperature and duration. Skin tends to hold heat, and the effect of charring clothing makes this worse. Therefore, cooling by the application of a stream of water is extremely effective in reducing the depth of burn.

Percentage of body surface burn

The effect of a burn on the body fluids depends on the percentage of the body burnt. The larger the area of the body that is burnt, the larger the number of

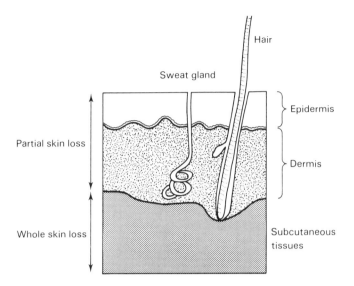

Fig. 30.1 Depth of burn.

capillaries that will be losing fluid. The fluid loss becomes significant if the burnt area exceeds 10% of the body surface of a child, or 15% of the body surface of an adult. A burn covering any area greater than these figures indicate will cause shock unless the fluid is replaced. The simple method of making a rough estimate of percentage body surface burnt is to use the rule of nine (Fig. 30.2). The surface area of the hand of the patient is about 1% of his body area, which is a useful guide. The head and neck make up approximately 9%, the complete leg 18%, the whole front of the trunk 18%, and the arm 9%. In a child, the head, neck and trunk are correspondingly larger, because of the small size of arms and legs.

Burns shock

Shock develops very rapidly, and the loss of fluid will continue for up to 48 hours. A third of the loss occurs during the first eight hours, so this covers the period of first aid treatment. Another factor during this early period is the emotional effect of the burn, which is often more severe in the smaller and painful partial thickness burns. The complications of burns are:

1. The complications of shock, and its effect on the organs generally.
2. Prolonged low blood pressure, which may lead to renal damage.
3. Sepsis. Early contamination with germs will cause an infection, and if this is severe it may invade the blood stream and produce septicaemia, a very

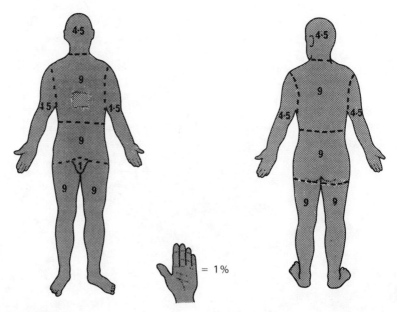

Fig. 30.2 Burns: rule of 9.

severe illness indeed. This is why every effort should be made to protect the burn from contamination during the early stages of first aid treatment.

Slow healing in a deep burn will cause scar formation: this may lead to gross deformities of the face and limbs. Early recognition of whole thickness burns enables the surgeon to excise the dead skin and replace it with a skin graft at an early stage. This will prevent shrinking of the skin or contractures.

First aid treatment of burns

Firstly, extinguish burning clothing and cool the burn. People whose clothing is burning tend to panic and rush around, which encourages the flames to spread rapidly. **Prompt action is required, to make the patient lie down and to smother the flames**. Use a jacket, blanket or any convenient piece of material and drop it straight onto the burning clothing, cutting off the air supply. Wrap the patient securely and then pour on water. The application of water is advised, both to cool the skin and to extinguish any smouldering cloth. Use running tap water for small hand burns: if possible, immerse the affected limb in cold water. Alternatively, apply wet packs (which will require renewing, as they tend to warm up). This will relieve pain and lessen the severity of the burn. Do not use ice water or place the whole patient in a bath.

Shock

The patient should be kept lying down and reassured. The patient will rapidly complain of thirst – this can be relieved by giving him fluids. The patient is unlikely to have an anaesthetic in hospital before the shock phase is fully under control, so there is no contraindication to giving fluids by mouth, particularly if the patient has to travel a long way to reach hospital. The oral route may well be the only method of replacing some of the lost serum. A teaspoonful of sodium bicarbonate plus a teaspoonful of salt in two pints of water will give a solution which can be drunk and which will replace some of the lost salts from the body. It can be made palatable with fruit juices. It must be emphasized that in cases of severe burns, the sooner the patient is moved to a hospital the better. If there are other injuries or if consciousness is impaired, oral fluids should not be given.

Maintenance of the airway

Patients with burns of the face, particularly if trapped in a burning building in which oil or modern furniture are burning, rapidly develop oedema of the face and respiratory complications from fumes. These patients need rapid evacuation to hospital for the insertion of an airway, and should be given first priority.

Prevention of infection

The burnt area is sterile from the effect of the burn. The process of irrigating with cold water even from a domestic tap is unlikely to introduce any additional infection. Where possible, the first aider should wash his hands and avoid touching the burn.

Dressing the burn

As a first aid measure for large burns, ointments and antibiotic creams should not be applied. Partially burnt clothing and smouldering clothing should be removed and a dressing laid on the burnt area. Burnt material stuck to the burn should be left. If available, sterilized non-adherent burn dressing of Gamgee and Melolin® (see Chapter 34) or the Roehampton® dressing of polyurethane foam (Fig. 30.3) should be applied. Failing this, freshly laundered sheets, pillowcases or towels can be used. The burn will exude a lot of fluid, so a thick layer of cotton wool is used, held in place with a crepe bandage.

Burns of the hand are treated by placing the hand within a polythene bag, loosely bandaging the wrist. This will enable the patient both to move his fingers easily and to avoid contamination. Where burns of the limb have also

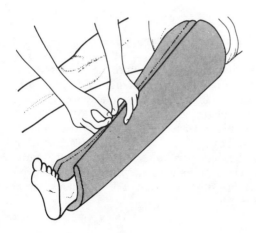

Fig. 30.3 Roehampton® Burns Dressing. Courtesy of Price Bros & Co Ltd.

occurred, the sterile dressing should be applied firstly to the arm, then the polythene bag placed over the hand. The limb may require splinting, but will in any case need elevation to avoid swelling of the fingers. Movements of the fingers can be encouraged.

Further medical treatment will be required, and where possible this is best done in the A & E Department of the local hospital. Priorities for treatment will be intravenous fluid for shock, then pain relief, and proper cleaning and dressing of the burn wound under surgically clean conditions in an operating theatre.

Advanced first aid treatment

There may well be circumstances in which early evacuation is not possible, e.g. at sea, on oil rigs, on expeditions in remote areas or with mass casualties. Under these circumstances the first aider may need to carry out the above regimen of treatment without medical advice being readily available. However, telephone or radio can be employed.

Follow the regimen as detailed above, giving priority to the fluid replacement for shock. The quantity of fluid given by mouth should be regulated hourly, measured and noted in a book. The quantity of urine that the patient passes should also be carefully measured, and the colour noted. The urine will be dark in colour at first, and fluids by mouth should be encouraged until the urine is more dilute.

Dressing of the burn wounds should not take place until the patient's condition is stable, with a normal pulse rate. With properly organized first aid kits, silver sulphadiazine cream should be available in all the above circumstances. This cream can be applied early to hands, face and burnt areas. Hands or feet can be placed in a polythene bag. A large amount of exudate will accumulate in this bag; it will require changing, for the first few days, at 24-hour intervals. Burns of limbs and body should be dressed with the burns dressing, a thick layer of cotton wool held on with a crepe bandage. This dressing should not be disturbed for several days. If the serum should start to ooze through the bandages, more cotton wool and more bandages should be applied on top of the original.

Special causes of burns

Friction burn. This is caused by sudden contact with a moving object – e.g. a road surface or lathe, or sliding quickly down a rope – where the heat generated burns the fingers. Treat as a burn.

Electrical burn. The heart beat or respiration may have stopped: this demands immediate action.

Cardiopulmonary resuscitation. See Chapter 5. Always switch off the electrical power before approaching the patient. Beware of high tension cables. Lightning burns are also electrical burns, and resuscitation will be the primary treatment required.

Chemical burns. Corrosive acids, alkalis, iodine and phosphorus will produce severe burns, as will lime (as found on building sites which is particularly dangerous). These burns should immediately be irrigated with copious amounts of running water, preferably continuously (e.g. from a tap) until all traces of the chemical are removed. If chemicals get into the eye, it should be irrigated under a running tap immediately. If the nature of the chemical is known, an acid burn should be irrigated with water to which bicarbonate has been added, and an alkali burn should be irrigated with a weak vinegar solution; but for chemicals in the eye, always use copious cool running water. The eye should be checked at the hospital as soon as possible. If any delay should occur in cases of lime in the eye, remove lime particles urgently by extra irrigation.

Sunburn. The sun and modern sun lamps are responsible for many burns. Artificial sunlight should be used with great care, and goggles always worn. These burns tend to be erythematous, but are painful. Calamine lotion is applied to ease the pain. A severe conjunctivitis in the eye often occurs with artificial sunlight burns. This is painful, with photophobia, and early medical attention is urgently required.

The first aid treatment of burns is simple and straightforward. Severe complications can be avoided by the efficient first aider. Seventy percent of burns which are kept clean will heal naturally. Mass burn casualties may be seen with many lightly injured survivors: efficient first aid treatment will save life and limb for many.

Nuclear Disasters, Chemical and Biological Warfare

NUCLEAR DISASTERS

It is horrific to realize that we are living in circumstances where nuclear explosions may happen, either through deliberate acts of warfare or due to an accident at, for example, a nuclear power station. It is important that the advanced first aider has some knowledge and understanding of the effects of these explosions.

Terminology

'**Thermonuclear**' **reactions** are those in which matter is destroyed and immense quantities of energy liberated. Such reactions take place constantly in the sun and other stars.

The power of thermonuclear weapons is measured by comparing them with the conventional explosive TNT. Thus a 1 kiloton weapon is equivalent to 1000 tons of TNT, and a 1 megaton bomb to 1 000 000 tons of TNT.

Nuclear weapons, however, produce many diverse effects which make them different in almost every way from even millions of tons of TNT.

Ground bursts and air bursts

A nuclear explosion on the ground is called a 'ground burst', whereas one at altitude is termed an 'air burst'.

An air burst would increase the area over which the explosion is felt but, relative to the ground burst, would have less effect immediately beneath the explosion. An air burst would also produce less local radiation but more extensive thermal damage (Fig. 31.1).

Radiation

Much of the energy released would be in the form of electromagnetic radiation, both above (ultraviolet, x-ray and gamma rays) and below (infrared and radio) the visible spectrum. The flash could cause blindness many miles from the explosion.

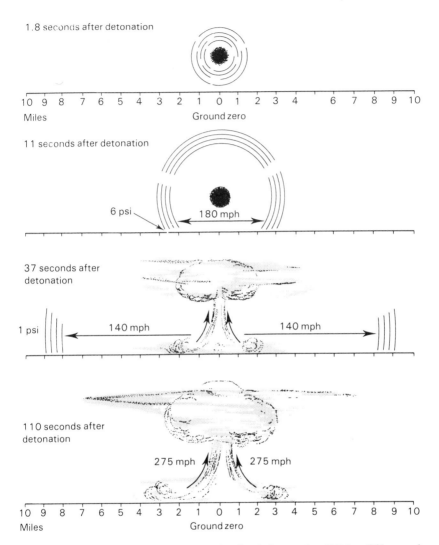

Fig. 31.1 Effects of blast from one-megaton nuclear bomb detonated at 6500 feet (PSI=pounds per square inch).

The heat given out would be such as to raise the temperature of the immediate area to millions of degrees Celsius. Any flammable material within three miles of the vaporization zone would be likely to ignite spontaneously.

The intense winds created by the explosion would blow at hundreds of miles per hour, and the ensuing firestorm would consume all available oxygen within its immediate area.

An 'electromagnetic pulse', resulting from absorption of gamma rays by the atmosphere, would severely disrupt radio communications, telex, telephone and computer equipment.

The exact nature and intensity of the radiation consequent upon a nuclear explosion depends on the exact characteristics of the bomb, where it is exploded, and whether it is a ground burst or air burst. Ground burst explosions suck huge quantities of dust up into the mushroom cloud, which then becomes radioactive. Many different chemical isotopes are produced. It is this radioactive material which returns to the earth as 'fallout'. Some of these isotopes may persist for hundreds of thousands of years.

Blast

The initial explosion would create a shock wave moving at supersonic speed. Buildings would be completely destroyed within a radius of several miles around the explosion of a moderate-sized weapon. People who were not killed by the blast might be fatally injured by flying debris from many miles away.

The medical effects of nuclear explosions

Many hundreds of thousands, or even millions, could be expected to be killed immediately by the blast over a moderate-sized city. A similar number would be severely injured. Many of these would inevitably die from the effects of hunger, disease, radiation sickness or further injury. There would be little shelter, no uncontaminated water or food and, in an all-out conflict, no neighbouring area is likely to be able to offer aid.

There could be panic, looting and general civil disorder. Modern medical services rely for their operation on sophisticated technology. In such a situation, skilled medical personnel would be little more effective than trained first aiders. Skilled first aiders would be able to give invaluable assistance to the large number of people with survivable injuries. Epidemics of diseases such as typhoid, cholera, hepatitis and dysentery could be expected. However, military experience has shown that even simple public health measures may make a significant impact on these epidemics. Disposal of the dead, however, remains an impossible task.

Radiation injury

This is divided into 4 types:
1. External whole body irradiation.
2. External contamination by radioactive material.
3. Internal contamination.
4. Radiation burns.

External whole body irradiation

A dose of radiation is measured in **rads**: acute radiation sickness develops at doses above 100 rads. Smaller doses may result in tumour formation in the survivors.

Three specific syndromes are described:

The neurovascular syndrome: this occurs after exposure to radiation levels greater than 3000 rads. It produces delirium, coma and convulsions and shock. Mortality is 100%.

Haematological syndrome. 450 to 1000 rads will affect the bone marrow and immune system. Death from anaemia and infection would be likely.

The gastrointestinal syndrome: 100 to 300 rads produce gastrointestinal effects such as vomiting and bloody diarrhoea. Mortality would approach 100% without facilities for intravenous fluid replacement.

Of course, these syndromes may overlap, making diagnosis difficult. The problem is further compounded by the fact that such patients may be difficult to differentiate from potentially salvable individuals with dysentery, malnutrition and dehydration.

Treatment would only be feasible for isolated occurrences, e.g. those which were the result of an accident, and in which help from adjacent areas – with full intensive care facilities – could be expected.

In the event of nuclear war it would be naive to expect to offer anything but the simplest treatment to mass casualties.

External contamination by radioactive material

The skin may be penetrated by radioactive particles (which may also be inhaled), or radiation may be absorbed from the body surface. The exact effect would depend upon the type of radiation (alpha, beta or gamma) being emitted.

Decontamination of mass casualties would be almost impossible.

Internal contamination

Inhalation or swallowing of radioactive fallout is likely. Again the effects would be dose-dependent.

Radiation burns

Local burns may occur from the absorption of high doses of gamma rays. These may be difficult to differentiate from classical (heat) burns and whole body irradiation.

The nuclear 'winter'

Fallout might be expected to occur for weeks, months or even years. Agricultural land and water supplies could remain radioactive for hundreds of years. Deaths from radiation sickness and disease would continue to occur and society would return, at best, to a mediaeval level, with hardly anything being able to grow. The dust in the atmosphere would shut out most of the sunlight, producing freezing temperatures and darkness for months.

Isolated nuclear accidents

These include such incidents as radiation leaks at nuclear power stations, or in fuel processing plants. Whole cities might be affected but, broadly speaking, uncontrolled nuclear explosions are extremely unlikely. The radiation leak is likely to take the form of radioactive gas, without a dust cloud or fires.

Protection of the population would be by evacuation of those settlements in the path of the gas. Under such circumstances the population would have all the support facilities of modern high technology medical care.

CHEMICAL AGENTS

These may be used in time of war or may be encountered through accidental exposure in industrial accidents.

The agents may be classified as follows:
1. Incapacitants.
2. Nerve toxins.
3. Blister agents.
4. Choking agents.
5. Inhibitors of cellular respiration.

Incapacitants

These agents produce temporary incapacitation of personnel. The disablement may last for hours or days. CS gas and tear gas fall into this group.

Nerve toxins

These are organophosphorus compounds like the insecticide parathion. They are rapidly destroyed by strong alkalis and bleach. Such agents inhibit the transmission of nerve impulses, which may produce paralysis and respiratory arrest. The time of onset depends upon the dose but may occur very quickly.

Immediate treatment consists of artificial ventilation and administration of atropine. Specific antidotes are available but need to be given early. Decontamination is important, as these chemicals can be absorbed through the skin.

Blister agents

These include 'mustard gas'. There is a delay between initial contamination and the onset of symptoms, i.e. the contaminated area shows redness and blisters form. The eyes and throat are particularly susceptible. Treatment is supportive, with decontamination and care of skin areas as in classical burns.

Choking agents

These cause acute inflammation of the lungs and pulmonary oedema (wet lungs). Phosgene is the best known example. Treatment is supportive, with oxygen if available and rapid transfer to hospital.

Inhibitors of cellular respiration

Various cyanide preparations may lead to such poisoning. Treatment is by artificial ventilation, preferably with oxygen.

In dealing with chemical contamination, care must be taken not to become contaminated oneself. This may be particularly difficult if artificial ventilation is required, unless resuscitation apparatus is available.

BIOLOGICAL WARFARE

Much experimentation has been carried out into possible means of disabling enemy populations using bacterial or viral organisms or their toxins. Various insect vectors, such as mosquitos and flies, have also been studied in this context.

The choice of agent would depend upon the circumstances of war. Agents with a high mortality, such as anthrax, might be used to inflict heavy casualties, but suspicion of biological warfare, outlawed by the Geneva Convention, would soon be aroused.

A more subtle approach, which might never be discovered, would involve the use of more 'usual' organisms, such as virulent influenza viruses or dysentery.

Biological agents, however, also present a risk to the aggressor in close geographical proximity. Natural or acquired immunity in the target population, and anticipation of attack, would render it much less effective.

Suitable organisms would need to be able to survive storage in a virulent state and be very potent to be effective after dilution in the air or in water supplies.

Some of the agents which might be considered for use in biological warfare are anthrax, botulism, cholera, various forms of dysentery, plague, typhoid, typhus, smallpox, influenza, encephalitis and other virulent viruses.

Personal protection depends upon a high level of suspicion, scrupulous hygiene and protection by suitable clothing. The armed forces possess special suits and respirators (NBC suits) for this purpose. Civilian populations, however, are very much at risk from inhalation of organisms in the air.

Pest control methods must be strictly enforced.

Most of the agents likely to be used will rapidly lose their virulence. Persistently virulent organisms would threaten the invading forces.

Decontamination by thorough washing in hot soapy water and burning of clothing is feasible. Buildings should be washed down with bleach and all water boiled.

Treatment of any established infection will be the normal medical management of the disease, including isolation procedures, immunization and antibiotic treatment.

32

Disorders of the Eye, Ear and Nose

THE EYE

Disorders of the eye, due to injury or disease, are very common and require careful and skilful treatment.

It must be clearly understood that the eye is the most delicate organ and even a slight injury is liable to be followed by unpleasant complications. Whenever possible, therefore, all except minor cases (e.g. foreign bodies under the eyelids) should be treated by a doctor.

Foreign bodies

Foreign bodies, such as insects and pieces of grit or metal, often enter the eye and may be quite difficult to discover. They produce a feeling of discomfort and grittiness, which is accompanied by redness, congestion and watering. These symptoms and signs are similar to those caused by disease, and if after a careful search the first aider fails to discover a foreign body, he must at once refer the patient to a doctor in case the trouble is due to a more serious condition (such as an ulcer).

Examination and treatment

The patient should be comfortably seated, with his head inclined backwards and suitably supported. The first aider should stand behind the patient and should examine the eye as follows:

1. Examine under lower lid. Instruct the patient to look upwards and, using the thumb, gently pull the lower lid down, drawing it away from the eyeball, so that its under surface can be examined (Fig. 32.1). If the foreign body is not found, it is probably under the upper eyelid, which must now be examined.

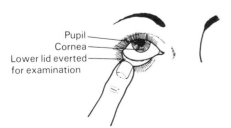

Pupil
Cornea
Lower lid everted
for examination

Fig. 32.1 Examination of the lower lid.

2. Examine under upper lid. This can only be undertaken when the eyelid is everted, i.e. turned inside out in such a way that its under surface is exposed. This process is painless and is undertaken as follows:

(a) Reassure the patient that he will not feel pain and instruct him to look downwards. It is essential that he should keep looking downwards throughout the examination.

(b) Place a match upon the middle of the upper lid, about 12 mm above its edge.

(c) Using the thumb and forefinger of the right hand, grasp the upper lid by its lashes and draw it slightly downwards towards the patient's cheek; then turn it upwards over the match, which is pressed backwards as the eyelashes are pulled up over it. The lid is now everted (Figs. 32.2 and 32.3).

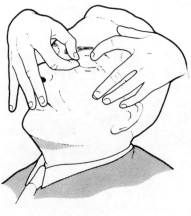

Fig. 32.2 Everting the upper lid (first stage).

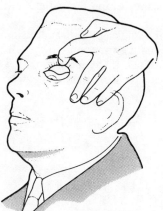

Fig. 32.3 Upper lid everted for examination.

(d) Instruct the patient to keep looking downwards. The under surface of the lid can now be thoroughly examined.

(e) When the foreign body has been removed, instruct the patient to blink; the eyelid will return to its normal position.

3. Remove foreign body. When a foreign body is discovered under either of the lids, remove it by touching it with a wisp of cotton wool or the twisted corner of a clean handkerchief which has been previously dampened with clean water.

4. After removal of the foreign body, the patient should be warned that unless his symptoms quickly improve he should seek medical advice.

Examination of the cornea

If examination of the under surfaces of the lids fails to reveal a foreign body, careful attention should be directed to the cornea, for a piece of grit or metal may be found sticking like a black spot to the front of the eye.

No attempt whatever should be made by the first aider to remove a foreign body which is adherent to the cornea, owing to the great risk of causing further injury. The eye should be covered with a pad and bandage to prevent movement and the patient should be referred to a doctor.

Attempts by those who are inexperienced to remove foreign bodies adherent to the eyeball may result in permanent impairment of sight.

Corneal abrasions

Scratches on the cornea, called abrasions, are caused by foreign bodies or by direct contact with rough objects (such as pieces of straw). They are very difficult to diagnose, but should always be suspected when a patient complains of the symptoms of a foreign body, although nothing is discovered on examination. These cases must be treated by the application of a pad and bandage, and medical advice must be obtained.

Failure to appreciate the possibility of a scratch on the cornea may result in scarring of the front of the eye and impaired vision.

Red eyes

Patients often seek the advice of a first aider because their eyes have become red and inflamed. The condition is frequently diagnosed by the inexperienced as a cold or chill, but the inflammation may be due to a more serious cause, such as ulceration of the cornea or inflammation of the iris, diseases which are quite beyond the scope of first aid.

It is best to refuse to attend patients suffering from red eyes, and to strongly advise the patient to seek a medical opinion.

Blows on the eye

Blows caused by squash balls and similar objects may have serious consequences, even when the lids are closed, because the delicate structures within the eyeball may be damaged or the back of the eye injured. The first aider should apply a pad and bandage and obtain medical advice as soon as possible, even though there may be little outward evidence of injury.

A common result of a blow is the well-known black eye, which is caused by bruising of the lids. A cold compress secured tightly in position by a pad and bandage will often prevent a black eye if applied early.

Perforating injuries

Occasionally, as a result of contact with a pointed object (such as a spike, dart, or a sharp branch of a tree), partial rupture or even perforation of the eyeball may occur. A small wound is usually visible and the pupil may become irregular. Sometimes part of the iris can be seen within the wound.

This is a serious accident and the patient should be kept lying down or be removed on a stretcher. His head should be kept as still as possible by placing sandbags at the sides. The eye should be covered by a lightly-applied pad and bandage.

Chemical burns

Burns of the front of the eye are common in industry and are usually caused by chemicals, e.g. lime, acids or alkalis. They may also occur in the home.

These burns are usually extremely painful and if permanent damage is to be avoided vigorous treatment must be started at once. Industrial first aid posts are usually prepared for this.

Treatment

Hold the head to one side so that the good eye is uppermost and will not be contaminated by the treatment. The lids should be separated with the first and second fingers of the supporting hand and the eye irrigated freely with copious amounts of running water from a spray connected to a tap or a large jug (Fig. 32.4). The head should be held over a wash-basin or bucket or the patient should lie on the floor. The irrigation should continue for at least ten minutes. After this treatment the eye should be covered with a pad and bandage and the patient sent to hospital.

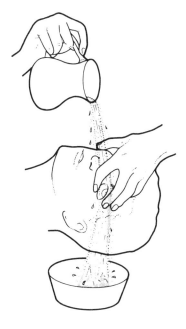

Fig. 32.4 Irrigation of the eye.

THE EAR

Four conditions liable to affect the ear are of interest to the first aider:
 (a) haemorrhage from the ear canal,
 (b) ruptured eardrum,
 (c) foreign bodies, and
 (d) earache.

Haemorrhage

Bleeding from the ear canal may be caused by a laceration, or may result from a fractured base of the skull, when the drum has been torn. The treatment of this condition has already been discussed (see Chapter 25).

Ruptured eardrum

This may be caused by, for example, a severe blow on the external ear, or a loud explosion. The condition is often accompanied by bleeding from the ear and by sudden deafness. The only first aid treatment necessary is to apply a light pad over the external ear, securing it in position by a suitable bandage.

The patient should be reassured and kept lying down until seen by the doctor.

A fracture of the base of the skull may be accompanied by rupture of the eardrum; hence a bloody discharge from the ear after a head injury is evidence of a fracture.

Foreign bodies

Foreign bodies in the ear may cause deafness due to blockage of the external ear canal. Occasionally a sharp foreign body may pierce the eardrum. This is a serious condition. Foreign bodies in the ear often become infected if they are present for a long time.

Treatment

1. DO NOT probe the ear with matchsticks, hairpins or anything else.
2. Try to remove insects with water run into the ear. (**Do not use cold water**, which will make the casualty dizzy; baby bottle temperature is about right.)

Do not pour water into the ear if the foreign body has been present for a long time, the casualty is deaf in that ear or the foreign body is sharp, in case the eardrum is perforated.

In any event, the ear should be examined at hospital or by the patient's own doctor.

Earache

First aiders are often consulted by patients suffering from earache. The trouble may be due to an abscess which, unless properly treated, may develop into an infection of the mastoid bone (at the back of the ear).

The first aider should strongly advise a medical opinion without delay, and will be wise to withhold treatment in order to ensure that a doctor is consulted. The pain is often relieved by adopting a sitting-up position.

THE NOSE

Three conditions liable to affect the nose are of interest:
- (a) fractures,
- (b) nose-bleeds, and
- (c) foreign bodies

Fractures

Fractures of the nose are generally caused by direct violence, e.g. blows. Pain, swelling and bruising are usually present; the nose may appear deformed and out of shape. Tenderness may be the only sign of a broken bone. In some cases the chief injury is internal, e.g. displacement of a delicate bone within the organ which may interfere with breathing.

A broken nose is a more serious injury than is commonly supposed, and often requires the services of a specialist for its treatment. The first aider should relieve pain by applying cold compresses and advise medical aid.

Nose-bleeding

This is usually venous in origin, and is occasionally serious; fatal cases have been recorded. Severe cases of haemorrhage are usually due to the rupture of a small vein in the nose.

Causes

There are many causes of nose-bleeding, classified as follows:

Injury. Blows on the nose may cause bleeding, and are sometimes associated with a broken nose. The possibility of the haemorrhage arising from a fractured base of the skull must, of course, never be forgotten.

High blood pressure. This occurs with advancing age and often causes severe attacks of nose-bleeding, which must then be regarded as one of the warning signs of stroke, though the bleeding may occur some years before an actual seizure.

Varicose veins. Small varicose veins are occasionally found inside the nose; these may rupture, causing profuse haemorrhage.

Altitude. Slight nose-bleeding occurs in susceptible subjects when a patient ascends to a high altitude, e.g. at winter sports or in mountain climbing.

Foreign bodies. Nose-bleeding, with discharge, in young children should always raise the suspicion that a foreign body may have been pushed up the nose.

Treatment

Reassurance. Loss of blood from any part of the body is always alarming, and for this reason the patient should be reassured that nose-bleeding is not dangerous and that the haemorrhage can soon be controlled.

Position. The patient should be comfortably seated in a chair with his head slightly forward.

Clothing. Tight clothing round the neck, chest and waist should be loosened to permit return of venous blood towards the heart.

Special instructions. The patient should be told to keep his mouth open and breathe through his mouth. He must also be warned not to blow his nose, which would dislodge any blood clot which had formed. Swallowing should also be avoided.

Warmth. The patient should be kept comfortably warm, but overheating may worsen the bleeding.

Pressure. The bleeding can often be controlled by firmly compressing the nostrils with the thumb and forefinger against the septum of the nose.

Medical attention. Medical attention is necessary to determine the cause of the condition and so prevent a recurrence: it will also be required for the more severe cases which do not respond to first aid measures.

Foreign bodies

Children often insert foreign bodies, such as buttons and beads, in their noses. Usually the accident is quickly discovered; the child itself calls attention to the fact that the foreign body has become lodged. Occasionally, however, the only clue to its presence is an unpleasant discharge from the affected nostril.

Treatment

Unless it is obviously easy to do so, the first aider should not try to remove the foreign body. The child should be prevented from touching his nose and should be told to breathe through his mouth. Removal of the foreign body may be quite difficult even for the doctor.

If the services of a doctor are unobtainable, the first aider must proceed with extreme caution. No attempt should be made to grasp the object, as it may be pushed further into the nostril and inhaled. The patient should be instructed to blow hard through his nose, keeping the sound nostril closed; he should be warned not to inhale through his nose before blowing, to avoid the danger of drawing the foreign body further upwards.

33

Bites and Stings

Animal bites (including human bites)

These may cause deep lacerations or puncture wounds which easily become infected. **Tetanus** may develop following deep puncture wounds.

In the UK **rabies** is not endemic, but in many countries, including the continent of Europe, it is prevalent. All live animals imported into the UK must undergo a period of observation in quarantine by law. Sometimes people attempt to smuggle their pets into the country. This is dangerous because rabies, once imported, will spread to wild animals (such as foxes) and through the population of domestic animals.

Rabies is a fatal condition in most cases.

A rabid animal is aggressive, drooling saliva and must be approached with care. If a case is suspected **call the police immediately**.

Treatment is available for those bitten by infected animals, but this must be given without delay.

If a bite is sustained abroad or from a suspect animal, the casualty must be transported to hospital immediately for treatment.

Snake bite

In the UK the only venomous snake is the adder (viper) (see Fig. 33.1) but zoos and private individuals keep other poisonous snakes in captivity. In countries where there are many venomous snakes, **identification** of the snake

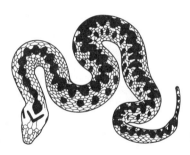

Fig. 33.1 Adder (*Vipera berus*).

279

is important to enable appropriate treatment to be given. If the snake has been killed, it should be taken with the casualty to hospital (if in a zoo, it can be identified on the spot).

Symptoms and signs

These depend to some extent on the particular venom, but general malaise, nausea, vomiting, confusion and difficulty with breathing and vision may be experienced. A shock state may develop. Small puncture wounds, usually two, may be visible at the site of the bite. As time passes, severe drooling of saliva may occur.

Treatment

1. Reassurance. Lay the casualty down.
2. If a limb is affected, immobilize it.
3. Call an ambulance immediately, stating that the casualty is a victim of snake bite.
4. Observe pulse, respiration and level of consciousness.

Insect and spider bites

Most insect bites and stings are trivial, but wasps, bees and certain spiders may be dangerous to some individuals. No dangerous spiders exist in the UK, but bites may occur from some species found in the south west of England.

Stings, including those of jellyfish and certain fish such as the weaver, may be very painful but are not usually a threat to life unless:
1. The individual is allergic to the venom.
2. Many stings are suffered.
3. The sting is in the mouth or throat causing swelling which may obstruct the airway, causing asphyxia.

Anaphylactic shock

Some individuals are so sensitive to foreign substances, such as the venom from an insect sting or a certain drug, that large amounts of the chemical histamine are released in the body. This causes swelling around the face and eyes as well as at the site of the sting, difficulty with breathing and rapid development of a shock state. **This situation may occur within minutes.**

Treatment

1. Call for an ambulance immediately.
2. Maintain an open airway.

3. Lay the casualty down; treat for shock.
4. Cardiopulmonary resuscitation may be required; monitor pulse and respiration frequently.

Bee and wasp stings

Following a sting, the poison sac and, in the case of bee stings, the sting itself will be left in the skin. It is essential to avoid squeezing the sac.

Treatment

1. Attempt to remove the sting with tweezers, if this can be done without exerting pressure on the sac. Use a magnifying glass if available to get a close up view.
2. Apply a cold compress.
3. If there is persistent pain or swelling, seek medical aid.

— 34

Bandaging, Dressing and Roller Bandage Techniques

THE TRIANGULAR BANDAGE

The triangular bandage is extremely useful in first aid. It is made by cutting diagonally a square piece of material 100–110 cm in length, so that two triangular bandages are formed.

Advantages

A triangular bandage is preferred to a roller bandage in first aid for the following reasons:
1. It can be used unfolded, or can be folded to make broad or narrow bandages.
2. It can be quickly and efficiently applied to any part of the body without moving the patient.
3. It can be easily improvised in an emergency from sheets and similar material.

Parts

To facilitate description of methods of bandaging, the triangular bandage is said to consist of four parts: the base, the point (or apex), the sides and the ends.

Uses

The triangular bandage can be used for many purposes, summarized as follows:
1. To secure dressings in position.
2. To form slings for the support of the upper limb.
3. To fix splints to the body or to a limb.
4. To secure pads.
5. A narrow bandage can be used as a roller bandage.

Securing ends

Reef knots are always used to secure the ends of a bandage, because they are reliable and can also be easily untied. Many students have difficulty in learning how to tie this knot, and several aphorisms have been devised to help beginners. In the method which follows it will be realized that the end which goes over first goes over again.

Method of tying a reef knot. Stage 1. Hold one end of the bandage in each hand, that in the right hand being slightly nearer the first aider's body than that held by the left.

Carry the end held by the right hand outwards (i.e. away from the first aider) and take it over, then under the end held by the left. Change hands and pull the ends tight, thus making the first loop of the knot.

Stage 2. Again hold one end of the bandage in each hand, this time, however, keeping the left hand nearer the body. (This, of course, is the end which went over first.)

Carry the end held in the left hand outwards over, then under that held by the right. Change hands and pull the ends tight to complete the knot.

The appearance of a reef knot is quite characteristic, and the ends of the bandage lie flat; in a granny knot, which is often tied by mistake (Fig. 34.1), the ends lie at right angles to the line of the bandage, even though an attempt may be made to hide this appearance.

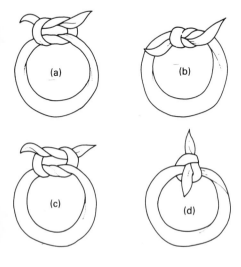

Fig. 34.1 A and B, reef knot; C and D, granny knot. Notice how the ends lie flat in the completed reef knot but across the bandage in a granny knot.

Surgeon's knot

This is a special kind of reef knot in which there is an extra twist in the first loop (Fig. 34.2). It allows a tighter reef knot to be applied.

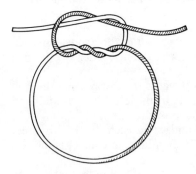

Fig. 34.2 Surgeon's knot.

Varieties of bandage

It has already been stated that the triangular bandage can be used unfolded, or folded to form broad or narrow bandages, as follows:

Broad bandage. A broad bandage is made from a spread-out triangular bandage by bringing the point down to the base and then folding over once.

Narrow bandage. A narrow bandage (Fig. 34.3) is made by folding a broad bandage once again.

Packing

When not in use, the bandage should be folded to make a convenient package as follows:
  (a) make the unfolded bandage into a narrow bandage,
  (b) bring each end to meet in the centre of the narrow bandage, and
  (c) double the bandage upon itself.
   It will be appreciated that if the bandage is folded by this method it can be quickly unfolded to made a narrow bandage ready for immediate use.

Use of the triangular bandage to form slings

Slings are used to supply comfort and support when an upper limb has been affected by an accident. Four kinds of slings are commonly used in first aid: the large, the small, the triangular, and the collar-and-cuff.

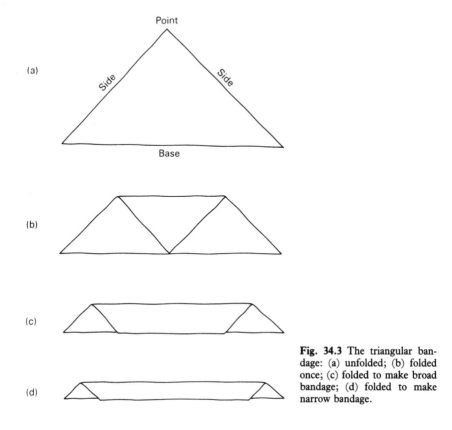

Fig. 34.3 The triangular bandage: (a) unfolded; (b) folded once; (c) folded to make broad bandage; (d) folded to make narrow bandage.

Large arm sling

A large arm sling is employed when both the elbow and the arm and forearm are to be supported. It is thus used for all wounds of the upper limb, fractures of the forearm and hand, and for broken ribs.

It should be remembered that when applying a large arm sling (Fig. 34.4) the point of the bandage must be placed at the elbow and the knot tied on the injured side.

Method

1. Place one end of an unfolded bandage over the shoulder of the sound side, allowing the remainder of the bandage to hang down the front of the trunk, with its point directed towards the elbow.

Place the point behind the elbow on the injured side.

2. Carry the upper end of the bandage round the neck so that it hangs downwards over the collar-bone of the injured side.

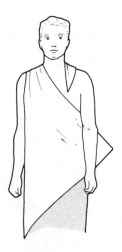 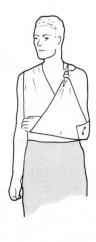

Fig. 34.4 Large arm sling (stages 1 and 2).

3. Bend the patient's forearm, keeping the thumb uppermost, until it is at right angles to the arm and rests in the middle of the bandage.

4. Collect the lower end of the bandage and bring it upwards over the forearm and elbow; tie both ends together in the hollow just above the collar-bone of the injured side.

5. Make final adjustments to ensure comfort; then bring the point of the bandage forwards to secure it to the front of the sling by the use of safety-pins.

Special notes

1. The forearm should be a little above the level of the right angle.

2. The fingernails should be left visible so that any change in their colour which indicates impeded circulation will be quickly noted.

3. The part of the sling at the back of the patient's neck can be placed under the collar of his coat, or even safety-pinned down to the back of his coat, to prevent discomfort.

4. The ends of the bandage should be neatly tucked away.

5. The sling should be free from wrinkles and creases so far as possible.

Small arm sling

This is intended to support the wrist and hand, while leaving the elbow free. The small arm sling (Fig. 34.5) is always made from a broad bandage, and the knot is tied on the injured side.

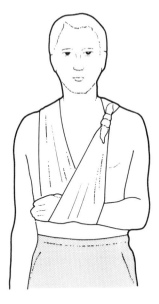

Fig. 34.5 Small arm sling.

Method
1. Put one end of a broad bandage over the sound shoulder, allowing the remainder to hang down the front of the trunk.
2. Carry the upper end of the bandage round the neck so that it lies over the collar-bone of the injured side.
3. Bend the patient's forearm until it is at right angles to his arm, with the thumb uppermost, and resting in the middle of the bandage.
4. Collect up the lower end of the bandage and bring it upwards over the wrist and hand; tie both ends together in the hollow just above the collar-bone of the injured side.
5. Make final adjustments to afford comfort.

Special notes
1. The support supplied by this sling should extend from the lower third of the forearm to the base of the little finger.
2. Twisting of the bandage at the back of the neck should be avoided.
3. Special notes 1 to 5 as described under large arm sling should be applied as far as possible.

The triangular sling

This excellent sling (Fig. 34.6) supplies great comfort to a patient, and is used whenever it is desirable to keep the hand well raised.

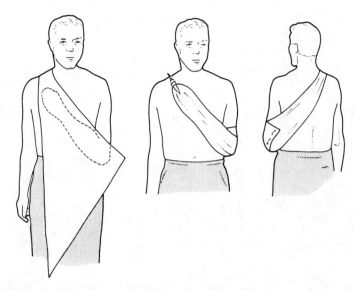

Fig. 34.6 The triangular sling: (a) first stage; (b) completed (front view); (c) completed (back view).

The chief point to remember when applying this sling is that the knot is tied on the uninjured side.

Method
1. Bend the patient's forearm so that his fingers just touch the collar-bone of the sound side. Provide support in this position.
2. Hold the point of the bandage between the forefinger and thumb of one hand, and one end of the bandage similarly with the other hand.
Apply the upper side of the bandage along, and parallel to, the upper border of the patient's forearm and hand, so that the point of the bandage extends a little beyond the elbow of the injured side.
3. Ask the patient or a bystander to support that part of the bandage which rests along the injured forearm.
4. Tuck the base of the bandage well under the injured forearm and hand.
5. Take the lower end of the bandage across the patient's back, over his sound shoulder, so that it appears on the collar-bone of the uninjured side. Tie the ends of the bandage in the hollow above the collar-bone.
6. Gently pull on the point of the sling to obtain freedom from wrinkles and creases and to ensure tautness of the bandage.
7. Collect up the point and tuck it under that portion of the bandage which is covering the front of the elbow.

8. Take the resulting flap of bandage to the back of the elbow and safety-pin it in this position.

Special notes
1. The usual remarks regarding position of knot, tucking in of ends, and freedom from wrinkles and creases apply in this as in all other bandages and slings.
2. It will often be found desirable to make a false point at the elbow before tucking in under 7. This can easily be done by turning in an extra flap from the lower border of the bandage which has been passed round the patient's back. The false point thus formed should then be in line with the point of the elbow.
3. Care should taken to prevent twisting of the part of the sling which crosses the back of the patient.

Collar-and-cuff sling

This type of sling (Fig. 34.7) is extremely useful in cases where it is desirable to restrict the amount of movement at the elbow joint. It can be made by forming a clove hitch (see Chapter 20) from a length of roller bandage. The hitch is placed round the wrist; the longer end is carried round the neck and tied to the shorter end in the hollow above the collar-bone.

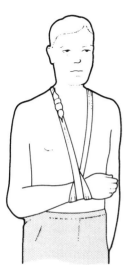

Fig. 34.7 Collar-and-cuff sling.

Use of triangular bandage to secure dressings

When practising these methods of bandaging, use a dummy dressing over the supposed wound and a sling when applicable.

Scalp: method

1. Fold in a hem along the base of a triangular bandage.
2. Place the bandage over the patient's head so that the point hangs down the middle of the back of the neck and the base is straight across the forehead (Fig. 34.8), just above the level of the eyebrows.
3. Take the ends of the bandage round the sides of the head, between the ears and the scalp, and cross them at the back of the skull. Finally, bring them back to the forehead again.

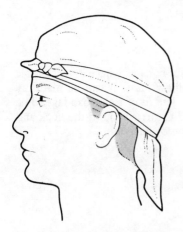

Fig. 34.8 Bandage for the scalp. Point of the bandage will be turned upwards to complete the treatment.

4. Tie the ends of the bandage on the base of the hem so that the knot is in line with the nose. Tuck neatly away.
5. Pull the point downwards to gain freedom from wrinkles and creases; then turn it upwards and safety-pin it in position at the top of the scalp.

Notes

1. The width of the hem governs the size of the flap at the back, which must be turned upwards at the end of the treatment. The point of the bandage should be fastened with a safety-pin in such a position that no discomfort is caused to the patient when he lies down.
2. The ends of the bandage must not be tied too tightly, or headache will result. The secret of applying a firm bandage to the scalp is to cross the ends at a fairly low level at the back of the head.

Eye: method

1. Place the centre of a narrow bandage over the affected eye. Arrange the bandage on the slant so that the lower end is inclined downwards and passes below the ear on the injured side, and the upper end passes upwards over the side of the head on the unaffected side.
2. Carry the ends round the head, cross them at the lower part of the skull and bring them forwards.
3. Tie the ends on the centre of the bandage (Fig. 34.9).

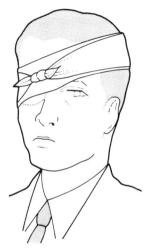

Fig. 34.9 Bandage to retain a dressing on the eye.

Notes
1. The bandage must be applied well on the slant to prevent obscuring the sight of the unaffected eye.
2. Some authorities do not like the knot tied over the eye itself and recommend that the bandage be finished off slightly to one side of the pad.

Forehead, side of the head, cheek or any part of the body that is round

A broad or narrow bandage applied in a manner similar to that for the eye should be employed, the ends being tied in a suitable position. Surplus bandage can be taken round a limb and tied.

Shoulder: method

1. Apply a small arm sling, arranging that the knot is placed along the course of a line drawn upwards along the midline of the outer side of the patient's arm into the neck (Fig. 34.10).
2. Place the point of an unfolded bandage under the knot and secure it temporarily in position, allowing the base to hang down the affected side.
3. Turn in a hem along the base of the bandage and take the ends round the middle of the arm; tie them on the lower border of the hem. Then safety-pin the point of the bandage over the knot of the sling.

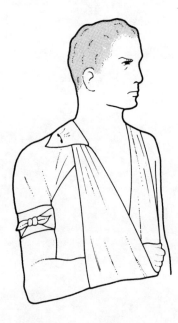

Fig. 34.10 Bandage to retain a dressing on the shoulder.

Notes
1. It is permissible to take the ends of the bandage twice round the arm, but care must be taken not to impede the circulation.
2. The two knots – i.e. of the bandage and sling – should be in the same straight line, e.g. along the course of the midline of the outer side of the arm.

Elbow: method

1. Turn in a hem along the base of an unfolded bandage.
2. Place the point of the bandage about 18 cm above the elbow (Fig. 34.11) on the course of the midline of the back of the arm.

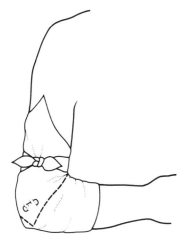

Fig. 34.11 Bandage to retain a dressing on the elbow.

3. Place the hem on the back of the forearm about 8 cm below the joint.
4. Collect up the ends of the bandage, carry them round the forearm, cross them in front of the elbow, and finally tie them about 8 cm above the joint, so that the knot is along the course of the midline. Tuck the ends neatly away.
5. Turn down the point over the knot and safety-pin to the bandage.

Notes
1. The commonest error is to turn in insufficient hem, which leaves too much point to turn down neatly.
2. If the bandage is applied with the elbow almost straight, then when the joint is bent (for example, to place the limb in a sling) wrinkles and creases will disappear, and the bandage will tighten. However, care must be taken not to impede the circulation.

Hand: method

1. Spread out a triangular bandage on a flat surface with the point directed away from the patient's body. Turn in a hem of suitable size.
2. Place the front of the patient's wrist at the middle of the hem, so that his middle digit is in line with the point and the injury is uppermost.
3. Carry the point of the bandage upwards over the back of the hand and forearm to a position about 8 cm above the wrist (Fig. 34.12). The patient can hold the point temporarily in this position.
4. Spread the ends of the bandage outwards to make two flaps, one on either side of the hand.

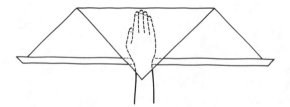

Fig. 34.12 Bandage to retain a dressing on the hand (first stage).

5. If the patient has a small hand, or the bandage is too large, fold each flap once upon itself.

6. Collect up the ends, cross them at the back of the wrist, and then carry them round the wrist to tie at the middle of the back of the joint.

7. Turn the point downwards over the knot (Fig. 34.13) and safety-pin to the bandage.

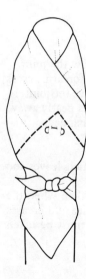

Fig. 34.13 Bandage to retain a dressing on the hand (completed except for turning down the point).

Notes

1. It will usually be found that a smaller hem than usual is desirable in the case of a hand bandage.

2. By keeping a slight tension on the point, wrinkles and creases can be avoided.

Wrist

This bandage (Fig. 34.14) can be used to retain a dressing on the palm of the hand; it is also useful for sprains of the wrist.

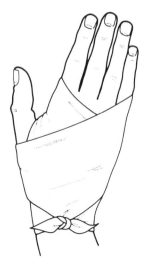

Fig. 34.14 Bandage for the palm of hand and wrist.

Method

1. Place the centre of a narrow bandage across the palm of the hand; collect the ends and carry them to the back of the hand, leaving out the thumb.
2. Cross the ends on the back of the hand and carry them round and round the wrist and lower part of the forearm; tie on the middle of the back of the limb.

Hip: method

1. Tie a narrow bandage round the lower part of the abdomen, so that the knot is on the injured side (Fig. 34.15).
2. Take an unfolded bandage and tuck its point under the knot, allowing the remainder of the bandage to hang down the thigh.
3. Turn in a hem along the base of the unfolded bandage and carry the ends round the thigh; tie them on the outer side of the thigh.
4. Turn down the point over the knot and safety-pin to the bandage.

Note: both knots should be in line with each other and placed along the middle of the outer side of the limb.

Knee: method

1. Place the point of an unfolded bandage about 18 cm above the level of the knee along the course of the midline of the thigh.

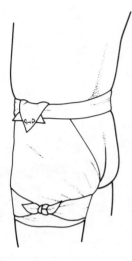

Fig. 34.15 Bandage to retain a dressing on the hip.

2. Fold in a suitable hem along the base of the bandage so that it now rests about 10 cm below the joint.

3. Collect up the ends, carry them to the back of the joint, where they are crossed and brought up to the middle of the front of the thigh, to be tied about 8 cm above the knee. Tuck the ends away.

4. Turn the point downwards over the knot (Fig. 34.16) and safety-pin to front of bandage.

Notes: see those for bandage of elbow.

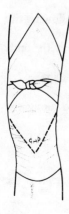

Fig. 34.16 Bandage to retain a dressing on the knee. Note: the point of the bandage will be turned down and safety-pinned to the remainder of the bandage.

Foot: method

1. Place the sole of the patient's foot on the centre of an unfolded bandage with the middle toe directed towards the point.
2. Bring the point upwards over the top of the foot to the front of the leg about 10 cm above the joint.
3. Smooth out the ends of the bandage to make two flaps, one on either side of the foot, as in the case of the hand bandage.
4. Bring the ends to the front of the ankle, cross them, then take them round the lower part of the leg. Tie the ends at the middle of the front of the limb about 5 cm above the ankle (Fig. 34.17).
5. Turn down the point and safety-pin to the remainder of the bandage.

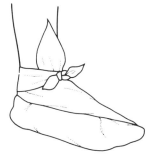

Fig. 34.17 Bandage to retain a dressing on the foot. Note: the point of the bandage will be turned down and safety-pinned to the remainder of the bandage.

Notes: it will usually be found that the use of a hem is undesirable in this bandage unless the foot is small.

The ends of the bandage should be tucked neatly away.

Ankle

This is sometimes used for the treatment of a sprained ankle, and is then made wet after application to make it tighter. Its use for this purpose is not very satisfactory, but if employed it should be applied over the shoe.

Method
1. Place the centre of a narrow bandage under the sole of the foot; carry the ends to the front of the ankle and cross them (Fig. 34.18).
2. Take the ends to the back of the ankle and cross them again. Carry them round the lower part of the leg and tie at the front of the limb.

Chest: method

1. Place the point of the bandage over the shoulder of the affected side of the chest, allowing the remainder of the bandage to hang down.

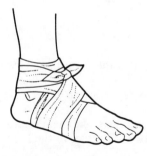

Fig. 34.18 Bandage for the ankle.

2. Fold in a hem of suitable size along the base of the bandage.

3. Carry the ends round the waist and tie them at the back of the affected side, leaving one end long and the other short.

4. Tie the long end to the point just behind the affected shoulder (Fig. 34.19).

Notes: both ends should be in line with each other at the back of the chest. The upper knot should not be visible from the front of the patient's body.

Back: method

1. Place the point of the bandage over the shoulder of the affected side of the back so that it touches the collar-bone, and allow the remainder of the bandage to hang down across the back.

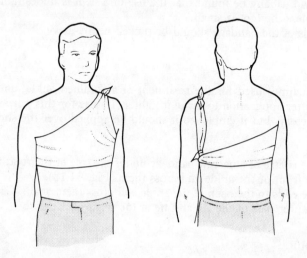

Fig. 34.19 Bandage to retain a dressing on the chest (front and back views).

2. Fold in a hem of suitable size along the base of the bandage.
3. Carry the ends round the waist; tie them at the front of the chest on the affected side, leaving one end long and the other short.
4. Bring the long end up to the point and tie in the hollow above the collar-bone (Fig. 34.20).

Notes: both knots should be in line with each other. The upper knot should not be visible from the back of the patient's body.

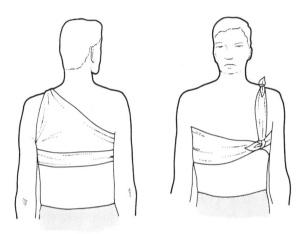

Fig. 34.20 Bandage for the back of the chest (back and front views).

Front of chest and abdomen

This part of the body can be covered by using two unfolded bandages.

Method
1. Place the base of a triangular bandage across the front of the patient's chest, allowing the point to hang down. Carry the ends of the bandage under the armpits and tie at the back of the chest.
2. Place the base of the second triangular bandage across the lower part of the abdomen so that it overlaps the point of the first bandage; carry the ends to the back of the body and tie together.
3. Tuck in the point of the second bandage under the base of the first and secure it in position with a safety-pin.

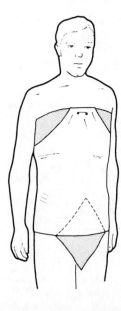

Fig. 34.21 Triangular bandages arranged to cover abdomen and chest.

4. Turn up the point of the first bandage over the base of the second and safety-pin it in position (Fig. 34.21).

Note. The above method is not very satisfactory, and whenever possible a roller bandage method should be used (see below).

Stump: method

1. Fold inwards a narrow hem along the base of an unfolded bandage.
2. Place the base of the bandage high up on the underside of the stump. Let the point hang down.
3. Carry the point upwards over the stump and there support it.
4. Cross the ends of the bandage in front of the point, then take them behind the stump and cross them again, finally carrying them forwards and tying in front.
5. Bring the point downwards over the knot and pin it (Fig. 34.22).

DRESSINGS

There is a wide variety of dressing materials available for covering wounds. It is useful to have some idea of their different characteristics so that the most suitable dressing can be obtained for the first aid pack.

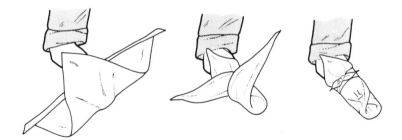

Fig. 34.22 Triangular bandage to cover an amputation stump.

The dressing has many functions. Its main purpose is to prevent wound contamination and damage to growing epithelium by avoiding friction and trauma. The wound will be less painful, and when there is a possibility of swelling, or the need to control haemorrhage, pressure can be applied. Wounds with a large amount of discharge will require an absorptive dressing. The less frequently a dressing is changed the quicker the healing process is. If the wound is comfortable leave the dressing until healing is complete, in 7–10 days.

All dressings placed in contact with wounds should be sterilized; there is no difficulty in obtaining these from a chemist. If possible, hands should be washed before dressing a wound. Neither the wound nor the part of the dressing in contact with it should be touched with the fingers.

Gauze

This is the simplest and most used dressing. It is both absorptive and protective, and is useful for all wounds. However, on raw abrasions and ulcers it tends to stick: when the dressing is changed new epithelium can be pulled off. Narrow ribbon gauze is useful for packing a cavity. Gauze should be 'fluffed up' to increase its absorptive capability.

Cotton wool

This can be used in dressing a wound as a layer over gauze to improve absorption or, when applied under a bandage, to apply pressure to the area. Rolls of thin cotton wool or cellulose material can be obtained, which are applied as easily as roller bandages and are very useful for sprains.

Gamgee tissue is wool between two layers of gauze and is very absorptive. Indeed, Professor Gamgee designed it for the purpose of dressing wounds with a lot of exudate.

Non-adherent dressings

Tulle gras is the oldest of these and is a fine mesh covered with vaseline, with or without an antibiotic. It is available in tins and is pre-sterilized. Tulle gras should applied one piece at a time and is very useful for small burns or abrasions.

Melolin® is a modern dressing. It consists of a layer of plastic film with micropore perforations covering thin layers of wool and gauze. This dressing is used extensively in hospitals; its advantages are that it does not stick, and any exudate will pass through the micropores into the wool.

A foam dressing, such as Synthaderm® is a modern synthetic skin used for burns, lacerations and ulcers, which works on the principle of keeping the wound moist and encouraging epithelium to grow rapidly (Fig. 34.23).

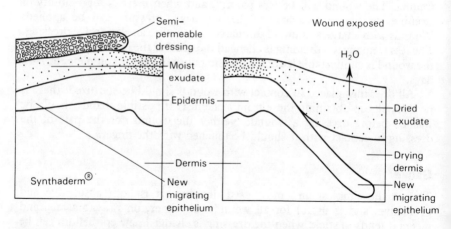

Fig. 34.23 Synthaderm®. Courtesy of Armour Pharmaceutical Co Ltd.

Transparent film dressings, e.g. Opsite® and Tegaderm®, are clear plastic dressings which are suitable for burns and abrasions. They do not stick to the wound, but the edges adhere to the surrounding skin. They also have the advantage of keeping the wound moist and encouraging epithelization.

Adhesive plasters and bandages

Zinc oxide strapping is firm and non-stretch, and has many uses in fastening dressings in place and reinforcing other forms of bandaging. As it is non-stretch, use with caution around joints and recently injured limbs which could swell.

Elastic adhesive BPC is the well-known elastic stretch bandage used extensively to give support and pressure, particularly for a recently sprained joint. Some people have sensitive skin, so it is best applied over a tubular bandage.

Plastic adhesive strapping BPC is a modern waterproof form of strapping.

Hypoallergenic tape, e.g. Micropore® is used in lieu of zinc oxide strapping for people who have sensitive skin.

Non-adhesive stretch bandages

1. Conforming bandage: minimum stretch but makes bandaging much easier.
2. Crepe BP: special weave with stretch.
3. Cotton crepe BPC.
4. Tubular cotton bandages with a special weave (e.g. Tubigrip®, Tubigauze®).
5. Stretch net (e.g. Netolast® and Surgifix®).

Roller bandaging

Although bandaging has been made very much simpler by the introduction of new forms of bandage, the art of applying a bandage is still necessary in first aid. Roller bandages are used for the following purposes:
1. To secure dressings to wounds: a conforming bandage is most suitable for this.
2. To exert pressure in the treatment of haemorrhage and varicose veins: for this purpose, a pad with a layer of cotton wool is applied under a crepe bandage.
3. To lessen swelling in the early stages of sprains and strains, and to support. An elasticated bandage applied over a layer of thin cotton wool is required, and either the crepe bandage or elastic adhesive bandage can be used. When a non-adherent bandage is required, the cotton crepe bandage BPC is slightly stronger and more firm than the crepe. A Tubigrip® bandage can be used if available.
4. To secure splints for fractures. A firm, non-elastic bandage is required and either domette (an open-weave woollen material) or unbleached calico is satisfactory.

Rules of bandaging

Never apply a bandage wet, as it will shrink and become too tight on drying. Choose a bandage of suitable width: 2.5 cm for thumb and fingers; 4–5 cm for the hand; 5–6 cm for the head, foot and forearm; 8–10 cm for leg, thigh and upper arm; 10 cm for breast or shoulder; and 15 cm for axillary or trunk bandages.

Skin surfaces should be separated by cotton wool with talcum powder to prevent chafing and soreness. When bandaging the axilla or groin, apply talcum powder and a layer of wool.

Bandaging

1. Stand in front of the patient on the same side as you are bandaging, looking over the shoulder. Exceptions: the capeline and eye bandage are applied standing behind the patient.
2. Support the part which is being bandaged in the position in which it is to remain, e.g. the elbow should be flexed to the degree required, the foot placed at right angles to the leg.
3. Learn to use both hands equally, changing the bandage from hand to hand as required, using the right hand for the left side of the body and the left hand for the right.
4. Place the outer side of the roll against the part being bandaged.
5. Start with an oblique turn downwards, so that the end of the bandage is firmly secured by the following turns.
6. Unroll the bandage, which should be in a firm roll, onto the part being bandaged; do not unroll it first and then put it on. This is most important, to ensure an even pressure.
7. Work from within outwards on the limbs, and from the injured side across the front on the head and trunk as a general rule.
8. Work from below upwards.
9. Cover two-thirds of the previous turn with each fresh turn, leaving one-third of the bandage uncovered.
10. Keep the turns parallel to one another.
11. Make the pattern lie on the outer side of the limb and keep it in one line. This will come of itself if the spacing and parallel line of the turns are good. Never make a reverse over a prominent bone.
12. Finish off securely with either a reef knot, safety-pin or special fastening. Never place the knot or pin over a prominent bone or a wound, and do not place it where it will cause pressure from the patient lying or resting on it.
13. To remove the bandage, loosen the end and pass the bandage from hand to hand over the front and back of the limb, gathering the loose bandage into the hands.

Patterns of bandaging

Many of the elaborate patterns used with the old calico bandages are not required with the new forms of bandage material but it is still necessary for the advanced first aider to become an expert. He should practice bandaging regularly, using different techniques. Opportunities should be taken to learn how to use the newer materials, which should be provided in first aid kits.

Pad and bandage

The field dressings and shell dressings, designed for war and used extensively in the field, have been adapted for civilian use and are now available in many sizes. A supply of these standard dressings, in varying sizes, should be always available in any modern first aid kit. The pad, with a suitably sized bandage already fastened (Fig. 34.24), is supplied ready sterilized in a pack. The pack

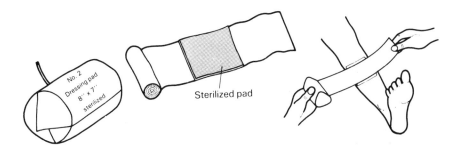

Fig. 34.24 Pad and bandage.

is opened by pulling the tab. When opening the dressing, it is important not to touch the face of the sterilized pad and to avoid touching the wound. The pad is placed on the wound and the bandage wrapped firmly around the limb. With large wounds, if this does not arrest haemorrhage, further pads then can be applied on top and held with the bandage.

Adhesive dressings

Small adhesive dressings (Elastoplast®, Band-aid®, etc.) can be obtained in a wide range of sizes, and they are highly suitable for many wounds that the first aider will have to treat. They are easily carried, easily applied, are comfortable to wear and have the advantage of being cheap. It is important that the wound is clean and that the surrounding skin is dry, otherwise the dressings will not adhere. Some of these are made of waterproof material which is useful for people at work. Non-adherent dressings with a perforated film of Melolin® are now available in various sizes; they are sterile, absorbent and easy to apply.

Patterns of bandaging

The circular turn, which is used on the head and trunk, the bandage going straight round the part.

The spiral bandage, with a slight upward slope, is useful for a limb where there is little increase in thickness, e.g. the finger and lower part of the leg.

The figure-of-eight bandage is also used for the part increasing in thickness; it is mainly used for the ankle and the hand.

The spica bandage is used for joints where one part makes an angle with the other, e.g. the hip, shoulder and thumb.

The recurrent bandage is used to cover an extremity, e.g. the end of the finger or thumb, a stump, the whole hand or foot.

There are also many special bandages used for parts of the head and trunk for which the first aider will often substitute the triangular bandage or the new materials.

The figure-of-eight bandage (for ankle or hand)

Start with an oblique turn across the affected part from within outwards, e.g. across the top of the foot. Carry the bandage across the sole at the base of the toes and up across the top of the foot, crossing the other turn and going round behind the ankle low down on the heel (Fig. 34.25). Bring the bandage over the top of the foot again and down towards the little toe, one-third of the width higher than the first turn; pass it under the sole and across the top of the foot to the back of the ankle one-third of the width higher than the first turn. Continue with foot and ankle turns until the affected part is covered.

The spica

A spica bandage is similar to a figure-of-eight, but one loop is very much smaller than the other. It is used for hip, shoulder and thumb.

The small loop encircles the thigh, arm or thumb respectively. The large loop encircles the waist, chest or wrist. It may be applied either as an ascending or descending spica (Fig. 34.26).

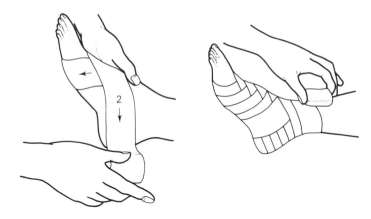

Fig. 34.25 The figure-of-eight to the left ankle begun (left) and completed (right).

For the ascending spica for the shoulder, start with an oblique turn downwards, working from within outwards, and carry the bandage round the arm and then up over the shoulder, across the back and under the opposite armpit; then carry it across the front of the chest over the shoulder and round the arm again one-third of the width of the bandage higher up the arm than the first turn. Next carry the bandage up over the shoulder and across the back to the opposite armpit, then back over the front of the chest, over the shoulder and round the arm again one-third of the width of the bandage higher up. Continue with alternate arm and chest turns until the dressing is covered.

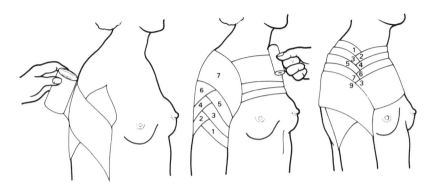

Fig. 34.26 Left to right: (a) ascending spica to the shoulder begun; (b) ready for fastening; (c) descending spica to shoulder completed.

For the descending spica, start with the turns high up in the armpit and high on the shoulder respectively. Work downwards one-third of the width of the bandage lower each time. It is better than the ascending spica when the wound is high over the shoulder.

For the hip, start with a loop round the thigh, working from within outwards; then carry the next loop round the trunk, and complete with alternate thigh and trunk turns, crossing on the outside of the hip.

For the thumb, start with a loop round the thumb, then carry the bandage round the wrist, and continue with alternate turns till the part is covered (Fig. 34.27).

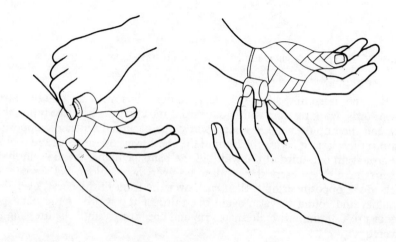

Fig. 34.27 Spica of thumb, begun and completed.

The recurrent bandage

The recurrent bandage is used for an amputation stump, the tip of the finger or thumb, or the whole of the hand or foot. Begin with a turn over the centre of the end of the part being bandaged; hold the turn with the thumb and fingers of the other hand. Fold the bandage back and carry it over the extremity to one side of the centre line covering one-third of the first turn. Again catch the bandage with finger and thumb, turn the bandage and bring it back on the opposite side of the centre turn, again covering one-third of the first turn and catch again. Now take a circular turn round the part to hold these previous turns, and repeat with another turn further out on either side, covering two-thirds of the previous turn; repeat if necessary and secure with another circular turn. Two or three turns on either side of the centre turn

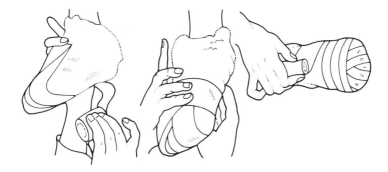

Fig. 34.28 Recurrent bandage applied to the foot, begun and completed.

suffice to cover the extremity, and the bandage is then completed with either spiral or figure-of-eight turns round the part (Fig. 34.28).

The capeline

This is used for fixing a dressing to the head. Take two roller bandages and sew or pin the ends together. Place the join in the centre of the forehead and carry the bandages round the greatest circumference of the head above the ears to the occiput. Cross the bandages here then turn one through 90° and carry it up over the centre of the top of the head (1) to the forehead (Fig. 34.29); carry the other straight on round the head and bring it over the first bandage at the forehead. Turn the first bandage back again over the top of the

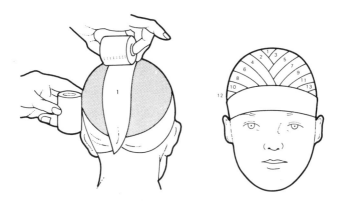

Fig. 34.29 Capeline bandage begun (left) and completed (right).

head slightly to one side of the centre line to the occiput (2), and again carry the other round the head and over the second at the back. Again turn the first bandage, and carry it back over the top of the head (3) slightly to the opposite side of the middle line; catch it by the other bandage at the forehead. Continue in the same manner, always using the same hand and bandage to go backwards and forwards over the head and, working outwards, leaving a third of the previous turn uncovered. Carry the other bandage round and round the head to catch and hold down the backwards and forwards turns of the first bandage. Work on till the bandages overlap well at the sides and the whole dressing is covered.

The eye bandage

Begin above the injured eye; carry the bandage horizontally across the forehead away from the affected eye and round the greatest circumference of the head. Cover half the turn again to the point behind the ear on the good side. Then carry the bandage down to the occiput and up below the ear and across the eye to the forehead; here either continue the same in line over the top of the head, down behind the opposite ear and up again over the eye, a third of the bandage further outwards, or make a reverse over the forehead and continue in the line of the first turn. As few turns as possible should be applied over the eye for lightness, coolness and ease of removal (Fig. 34.30). If a reverse is made it can be held with a long ordinary pin threaded in and out, with head uppermost. It will not slip out and prevents the patient from fumbling with the bandage.

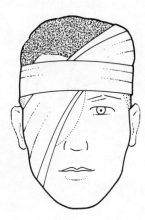

Fig. 34.30 The eye bandage, completed.

The 'T' bandage

This is used to fix dressings over the perineum. It consists of two strips of material each about 13 cm wide (Fig. 34.31). One is folded over and made into a waist belt (this must be long enough to tie round the waist). The second is fixed into the centre of the belt at the back like the downstroke of the letter 'T', and the edges are hemmed. It is divided up into two tails at the other end, leaving about 25 cm undivided.

To apply, tie the waist belt in position comfortably. Bring the other piece between the thighs and up over the abdomen and secure to the waist belt, crossing the tails to the opposite side.

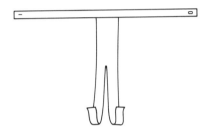

Fig. 34.31 Pattern of the 'T' bandage.

Tubular gauze bandaging

Tubular gauze is now quite widely used and may be encountered by the first aider. It consists of a woven cotton bandage prepared in the form of a tube, which is applied over the part to be bandaged by means of a special applicator. It is available in several sizes, suitable for bandaging all parts of the body from individual fingers to the entire trunk. Tubular applicators of appropriate diameter are provided for all but the largest sizes, although any size of the material can be applied without them. Tubular gauze is more quickly and easily applied than are roller bandages (particularly when treating the limbs and head), and its chief use is for securing dressings in place without restricting the movement of the limb or part. Tubigrip® which uses an elastic weave (Fig. 34.32), is used to apply pressure and also give support for soft tissue injuries.

Elastic adhesive bandage (EAB)

The ankle. Use 7.5 cm or 10 cm Elastoplast EAB (depending on the size of the limb).

The foot is held dorsiflexed and everted for a lateral sprain and dorsiflexed and inverted for a medial sprain (Fig. 34.33).

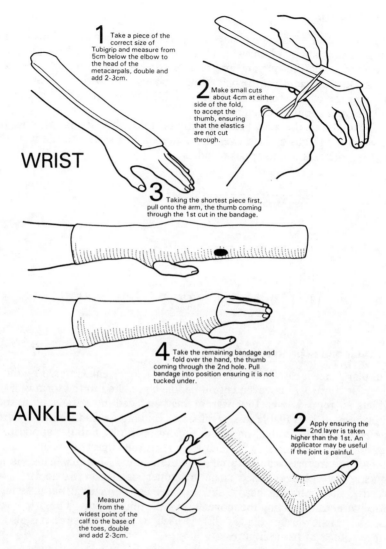

Fig. 34.32 Bandaging using Tubigrip®: (a) wrist; (b) ankle. Courtesy of Seton Products Ltd.

Attach the Elastoplast bandage at the base of the toes. For a lateral sprain start on the top of the foot and work from the outside to the inside to keep the foot in eversion. For a medial sprain start on the inside and work outwards. In almost all cases the bandage is started at the joint below the injury and worked upwards.

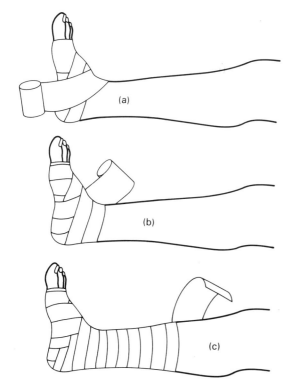

Fig. 34.33 Ankle bandaging using Elastoplast® EAB. Courtesy of Smith & Nephew Medical Ltd.

Take two fixing turns around the foot and then bring the bandage down at an angle to take one turn around the heel. Using moderate tension, continue in a figure-of-eight fashion over the dorsum of the foot (A), round the back of the heel, over the dorsum of the foot and under the heel, for three or four complete turns (B).

Each turn should overlap so that the bandage proceeds from the heel towards the toes and up the back of the heel towards the ankle.

Still using moderate tension, bandage up the leg, overlapping by about half, to finish just below the knee (C).

Thumb and thenar muscle injuries

The basic principle when dressing the thumb is to follow a series of figure-of-eight turns.

Techniques. Use 2.5 cm Elastoplast Plaster.

Starting below the distal interphalangeal joint, with the back of the hand uppermost, apply two turns around the thumb (On the left thumb turn anti-clockwise, on the right thumb turn clockwise) (Fig. 34.34(a)).

Bring the plaster straight across the palm, around the hand and over the base of the thumb.

Continue into the cleft of the thumb, around the thumb itself and back again across the palm (Fig. 34.34(b)).

Repeat the entire sequence for three or four complete turns, overlapping each turn by at least half to work down the thumb and down the palm towards the wrist (Fig. 34.34(c)).

Then take one further layer across the base of the palm and finish with two or three complete turns around the wrist (Fig. 34.34(d)).

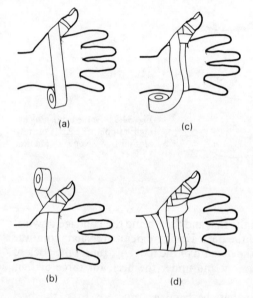

(a)

(c)

(b)

(d)

Fig. 34.34 Thumb bandaging using Elastoplast® Plaster. Courtesy of Smith & Nephew Medical Ltd.

It is important to check the circulation distal to the bandage by pressing the nail and watching the colour return. If there is evidence that the bandage is too tight, it should be removed.

Finger injuries

This simple method is appropriate for sprains, reduced dislocations of the fingers and for **stable** fractures of the phalanges and metacarpals.

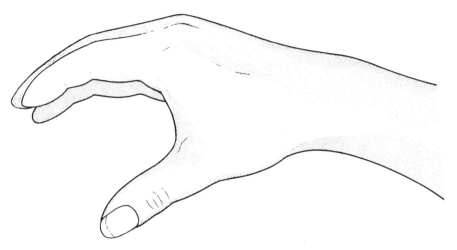

Fig. 34.35 'The "safe" position of the hand.'

Note that two skin surfaces should not be bandaged together unless a pad of absorbent material is first placed between them to prevent sores occurring. The fingers should be bandaged so that interphalangeal joints are straight, as shown in Fig. 34.35.

Technique. Use 2.5 cm Elastoplast Plaster and a small piece of gauze.

Position the piece of gauze between the injured finger and the one next to it. Then apply two lengths of Elastoplast Plaster, approximately 20 cm long, around both fingers, leaving the interphalangeal joints free (Fig. 34.36).

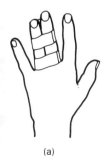

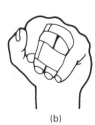

(a)   (b)

Fig. 34.36 The use of Elastoplast® Plaster for sprains, reduced dislocations of the fingers and the stable fractures of the phalanges and metacarpals. Courtesy of Smith & Nephew Medical Ltd.

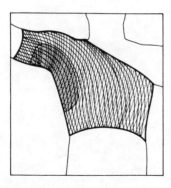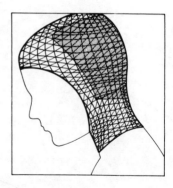

Fig. 34.37 Elastic net bandages. Courtesy of Seton Products Ltd.

Elastic net bandages

These are extremely useful for holding dressings in difficult places where other methods are not possible. In hot weather they avoid the hazards of sweating and skin reaction to strapping. A range of these dressings (Netolast®, Surgifix®, etc.) is obtainable, and they are recommended for the advanced first aider's pack (Fig. 34.37).

Wound dressings and bandages have been used for many thousands of years: the materials may differ but they will be required in first aid for the next millennium.

35

Transport of the Sick and Injured

GENERAL PRINCIPLES

Rescue

In accidents, the victim may be trapped in wreckage or debris. In such cases the first aider must decide whether or not the patient should be removed before first aid is given. This will depend upon the need to give life-saving attention. In many cases it will be less disturbing to the patient if he is left until rescue services with adequate equipment arrive. At all times it is the comfort and welfare of the patient which must be considered. Anything which might worsen injuries or increase shock must be avoided. Transport of the sick and injured is an important branch of first aid; much may depend on the careful manner in which a patient is removed to shelter after an accident.

The two methods of transport are manual or by stretcher.

Manual methods

These include all methods of carrying a patient by hand. They are suitable for moving a patient for a short distance, e.g. off a football field. Their great advantage is that they can be undertaken by one or two helpers. Except in an emergency, they should not be used for patients who have been seriously injured.

Manual methods can be divided into two categories:
1. Support by a single helper.
   - (a) the cradle carry
   - (b) the human crutch
   - (c) the pick-a-back
   - (d) dragging
   - (e) the drag carry
   - (f) fireman's lift and carry.
2. Support by two helpers.
   - (a) the two-hand seat.
   - (b) the human stretcher
   - (c) the three-hand seat
   - (d) the four-hand seat
   - (e) the fore-and-aft carry.

Stretcher methods

These include stretcher-bearing and the use of ambulances. They are more satisfactory than manual methods and should be used for all serious cases such as shock, haemorrhage, and fractures of the spine, pelvis and lower limbs.

Four helpers are necessary for stretcher-bearing if the journey is a long one; shorter journeys can be undertaken by two bearers. Whenever possible, however, long journeys should be avoided. In England, it is usually possible to obtain an ambulance within a short space of time. Hence it is often wise, if the case is serious, to remove the patient on a stretcher to a temporary shelter where he can await the arrival of the ambulance, thus avoiding a long journey by stretcher.

Rules for transport

Whichever method of transport is adopted, it must fulfil the following conditions:

Safety. It hardly seems necessary to mention that transport must be safe. However, cases have occurred in which patients have fallen off a stretcher or the stretcher itself has become unserviceable and collapsed. Stretchers should be inspected periodically.

Steadiness. Transport must be steady and great care must be taken to avoid jolting or jarring the patient.

Speed. The patient must be removed as quickly as possible provided that safety and steadiness are preserved. Sometimes, for example, it is necessary to drive an ambulance slowly and to sacrifice speed to provide comfort and safety.

Observation. The patient must be kept under continuous observation throughout the removal. Dressings must be examined to see that they remain securely fixed and that there is no recurrence of bleeding. Constrictive bandages must be readjusted at intervals and the patient should be watched carefully to make certain that there is no change for the worse in his condition.

SUPPORT BY A SINGLE HELPER

The cradle carry

This is valuable for carrying children and patients who are light; it cannot be used for those who are heavy (Fig. 35.1).

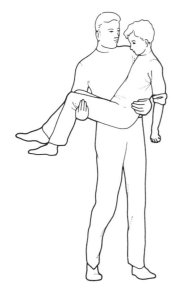

Fig. 35.1 The cradle carry.

Method. The first aider stoops by the side of the patient, places one arm under his knees and the other well round his back, rises (using the power of his legs) and carries the patient.

The human crutch

This can be used for a patient who is suffering from a slight injury to one leg only, e.g. a sprained ankle. The patient must be able to help by placing light weight on the injured foot and by supporting himself against the first aider's body (Fig. 35.2).

Method
1. The first aider stands on the injured side of his patient, places his near arm round the waist, and grasps some of the clothing on the sound side of the patient's body near his hip.
2. He instructs the patient:
    (a) to place his near arm round his neck so that his hand can be supported;
    (b) to march out of step with the first aider, beginning with the injured foot; and
    (c) to throw his weight onto the first aider as the patient takes each step with his injured foot.

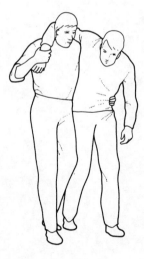

Fig. 35.2 The human crutch.

3. Using his free hand, the first aider grasps and supports that of the patient.
4. The patient tends to fall away from the first aider as they walk; to prevent this the first aider should pull the patient slightly towards him each time the sound foot is on the ground.

Pick-a-back

This well-known method can be used if the patient is conscious and able to support himself on the first aider's back (Fig. 35.3). When carrying by the

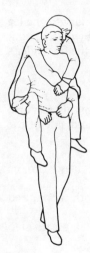

Fig. 35.3 The pick-a-back.

pick-a-back method, always try to clasp your hands. This will assist you when carrying the patient.

Dragging

This is used to remove an unconscious patient for a short distance, e.g. away from machinery or from a burning room. The patient should be turned onto his back; the first aider stoops behind his head, facing his feet, places his hands under the patient's armpits and walks backwards.

To drag a patient down a staircase, the first aider should crawl backwards down the stairs, supporting the patient's head upon his chest. When time permits, the patient's hands should be tied together on the front of his chest before dragging is begun.

The drag carry

This is an alternative to simple dragging, and is valuable for removing an unconscious patient from a burning room or from a confined space which does not permit the first aider to stand upright.

Method
1. The patient should be placed on his back and his wrists tied together.
2. The first aider kneels astride his patient and threads his neck through the loop made by the tied wrists.
3. By crawling forwards on his hands and knees, the first aider can drag his patient to safety.

The fireman's lift and carry

This is a useful method of carrying a patient who is unable to walk, but must only be used when the patient is not too heavy for the first aider. It has the advantage of leaving the first aider one free hand (Fig. 35.4).

Method. The first aider lifts the patient into the upright position and grasps the patient's right wrist with his left hand; then, bending down with his head under the patient's extended right arm, places his right arm round or between the patient's legs. Taking the weight on his right shoulder he rises to the erect position and pulls the patient across both shoulders, transferring the patient's right wrist to his right hand, so leaving the first aider's left hand free.

SUPPORT BY TWO HELPERS

These methods consist chiefly of the hand-seats which are used to carry patients when a stretcher is not obtainable. By these methods a patient can be

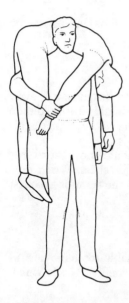

Fig. 35.4 The fireman's lift and carry.

carried for a short distance efficiently, but it is difficult to maintain steady transport.

In all two-helper methods (except the fore-and-aft carry) the helpers must walk out of step, beginning with their feet which are furthest away from the patient. They should keep their knees slightly bent to avoid jolting the patient and march with cross-over and not short side-steps.

The two-hand seat

This is used to carry a patient who is unable to use his arms. He must, however, be conscious and be able to keep his body erect (Fig. 35.5).

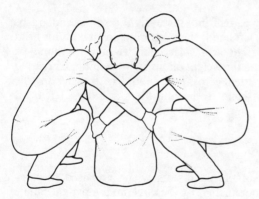

Fig. 35.5 The two-hand seat: preparing to lift.

Method
1. The patient should be placed in the sitting position.
2. The two helpers stoop, facing each other, one on either side of the patient's body. They must not kneel, because they would have difficulty in rising again.
3. Each helper now places his arm which is nearest to the patient's head across his back and grasps some of the clothing on the opposite side of the patient's body. Thus the helpers have crossed arms behind the patient's back.
4. The helpers raise the patient slightly with their crossed arms, and then pass their free forearms under the middle of his thighs, where they clasp hands by a special method called the hook grip (Fig. 35.6), which is made as follows:

The helper on the left side of the patient keeps his palm upwards and holds a folded handkerchief in his hand to prevent discomfort caused by the fingernails of his colleague.

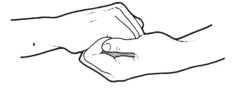

Fig. 35.6 The hook grip.

The helper on the right grasps his colleague's hand, keeping his palm downwards.
5. Both helpers rise together, raising the patient between them (Fig. 35.7).

The human stretcher

This is a very valuable method of carrying a patient in the lying-down position, and can be used for unconscious cases (Fig. 35.8).

Method
1. The helpers face each other, one on either side of the patient, and stoop beside him.
2. Each helper places his left hand under the patient's hips and clasps that of his colleague, by the hook grip mentioned above (see Fig. 35.6).
3. The helper with a free hand near the patient's head places his arm under the head, neck and shoulders, which must be carefully supported.

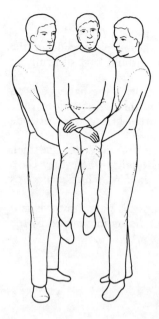

Fig. 35.7 The two-hand seat: ready to advance.

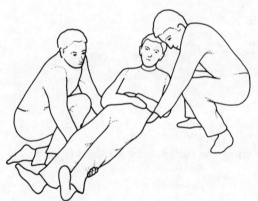

Fig. 35.8 The human stretcher: preparing to lift.

4. The helper with a free hand near the feet places his wrist and hand under the calves.

5. The helpers rise and carry the patient (Fig. 35.9).

Three-hand seat

This is used to carry a patient who is able to assist by using his arms. It is designed to supply support for one or both of the lower limbs during transport (Fig. 35.10).

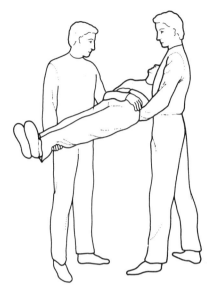

Fig. 35.9 The human stretcher: ready to march.

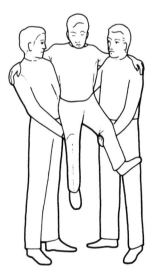

Fig. 35.10 The three-hand seat with hook grip.

Method

1. The patient should be placed in the sitting position.
2. The helpers stoop, facing each other, one on each side of the patient.
3. The patient is told to place his arms round the helpers' necks and to raise himself slightly from the ground so that a seat can be formed under him.

4. The helper on the injured side places his hand which corresponds to that of the injury under the calf or thigh of the affected limb. Hence he has one hand free to make a seat for the patient.

5. A suitable seat is formed under the patient as follows:

The helper with both hands free clasps his own left wrist with his right hand.

The helper who has one arm free interlocks his hand with that of his colleague by clasping his free wrist and allowing his own to be grasped.

6. Both helpers rise together, keeping the injured limb well supported.

Four-hand seat

This can be used when the patient is able to assist by using one or both of his arms and does not require support for either of his lower limbs (Fig. 35.11).

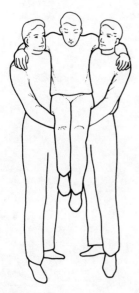

Fig. 35.11 The four-hand seat.

Method

1. The patient should be in the sitting position.
2. The helpers stoop, facing each other, on opposite sides of, and slightly behind, the patient's body.
3. The patient is instructed to place his arms round the necks of the helpers and raise himself slightly from the ground.

4. A seat is formed under the patient as follows:

Each helper grasps his left wrist with his own right hand, keeping the palms downwards.

The helpers interlock their hands under the patient, each grasping his colleague's right wrist with his left hand.

5. The helpers rise together, lifting the patient (Fig. 35.12).

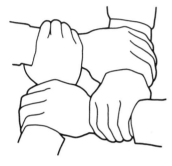

Fig. 35.12 Four-hand seat: position of the bearers' hands.

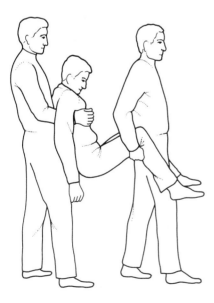

Fig. 35.13 The fore-and-aft carry.

Fore-and-aft method

This must be undertaken when space does not permit the use of ordinary hand seats. It is invaluable for removing a patient through a door or along a narrow corridor, but otherwise the method is not satisfactory, because it is uncomfortable and may cause difficulty in breathing (Fig. 35.13).

Method

1. The first helper stoops behind the patient's back and passes his hands under the armpits, clasping his hands together at the front of the chest.
2. The second helper places himself in front of and between the patient's legs with his back to the patient. He stoops and grasps the legs above the knees so that the legs are on either side of his body.

   If the patient is a woman, or when both legs have been injured, the limbs can be tied together and carried under the arm.
3. Both helpers rise together and walk in ordinary steps.

— 36

Transport by Stretcher

Standard stretchers

The Furley stretcher

There are many varieties of stretchers, but those most recommended by ambulance organizations are named after the late Sir John Furley. They are robust and cheap and are easy to fold, store and set up for use. Millions have been used throughout the world, and it seems likely to remain the general purpose stretcher (Fig. 36.1).

Stretchers are usually stored and carried in the closed position. To close a stretcher, the traverses should be bent at their joints so that the poles come together. The canvas bed is neatly folded and the slings laid along each pole

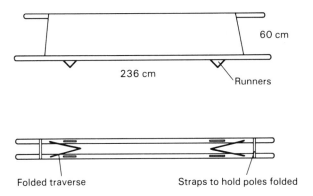

Fig. 36.1 Furley stretcher.

so that their buckles are at opposite ends of the stretcher; the transverse straps are taken round the canvas and the poles are fastened so that the stretcher is securely closed.

The telescopic

This is very similar to the ordinary stretcher, except that the handles can be slid under the poles, thus reducing its length to 6 feet. A telescopic stretcher is valuable for use in a confined space or when a patient has to be carried up or down a staircase.

There are many modifications of the standard stretcher, designed for special circumstances. Each has disadvantages as well as advantages. When making first aid plans for hazardous sports, the type of stretcher should be carefully selected. Some of these special stretchers are briefly described below.

Note. It is advisable, when arranging first aid cover for an event, to ensure that your stretcher will fit the ambulances which are likely to evacuate casualties. Attachments are made for stretchers which will take a transfusion bottle or elevate a fractured limb.

Stretcher poles and carrying sheets

Stretcher canvases are ideal for moving patients easily, and once the patient has been placed on one he is not disturbed by further changes. Subsequent moves are made by reinserting the stretcher poles. These canvases are ideal for laying on stretchers or beds in first aid stations (Fig. 36.2).

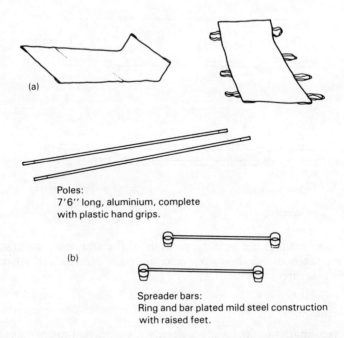

(a)

Poles:
7'6" long, aluminium, complete
with plastic hand grips.

(b)

Spreader bars:
Ring and bar plated mild steel construction
with raised feet.

Fig. 36.2 Stretcher poles and carrying sheets. Courtesy of FW Equipment Co Ltd.

Emergency stretchers

Modern materials are used to produce a modified Furley stretcher which is robust and stores easily. The hinged variety is ideal for carrying to all sporting activities (Fig. 36.3).

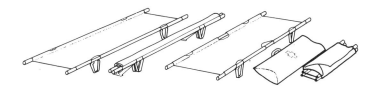

Fig. 36.3 Emergency stretchers. Courtesy of FW Equipment Co Ltd.

Scoop stretcher

The use of this stretcher has been described in Chapter 22 (Fig. 36.4). It is of value in cases of multiple injuries; the patient does not have to be unduly disturbed as the stretcher is moved and fixed under him. Traction applied to an injured limb will make it easier to close the stretcher.

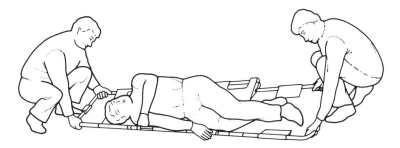

Fig. 36.4 Scoop stretcher. Courtesy of FW Equipment Co Ltd.

Flectalon® – Rescue stretcher blanket

This is a combined carrying sheet and body heat retaining blanket, designed for carrying patients from places with a risk of hypothermia. The blanket has carrying angles, and is made of a tough fabric with a thermal reflective insulation (which acts even under wet conditions). It is ideal for mountain or cave rescue (Fig. 36.5).

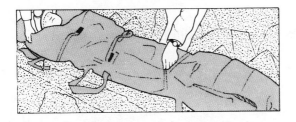

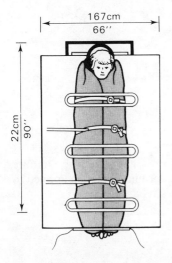

Fig. 36.5 Flectalon® rescue stretcher blanket. Courtesy of FW Equipment Co Ltd.

The Neil Robertson stretcher

This stretcher, made of strips of wood, canvas and rope, fits the body closely and has a general splinting effect (Fig. 36.6).

It is used for removing casualties from confined spaces or difficult situations from which the patient has to be lowered or lifted (Fig. 36.7).

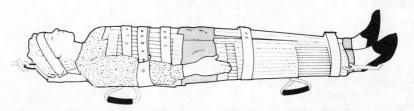

Fig. 36.6 The Neil Robertson stretcher in use. Courtesy of FW Equipment Co Ltd.

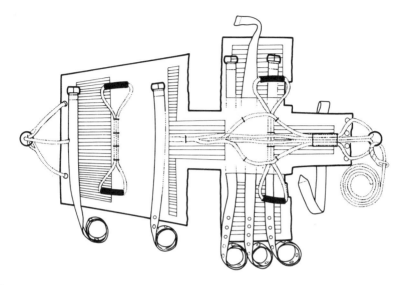

Fig. 36.7 The Neil Robertson stretcher. Courtesy of FW Equipment Co Ltd.

The Paraguard rescue stretcher

A light metal close-fitting stretcher with plastic cushioning (Fig. 36.8). It too is excellent for use in confined spaces, and has the added advantage that it can be made flexible in the middle for negotiating narrow corners, as in the rescue of injured pot-holers (Fig. 36.9). It can also be folded for compact storage and carriage (Fig. 36.10).

The vacuum stretcher

This is a soft, water-resistant cover full of minute polythene granules (Fig. 36.11). The patient is laid into this and the stretcher gently moulded around him. The application of a vacuum converts this into a rigid support which enables him to be moved easily and quickly (Fig. 36.12). These are popular on the Continent in helicopter rescue. They are robust, with smooth walls to protect the patient. Runners under the basket enable the stretcher to slide over rough spots.

Ambulance trolleys

These trolleys usually take the form of a telescopic stretcher on wheels, which normally has an anti-roll mattress to give additional stability during transport.

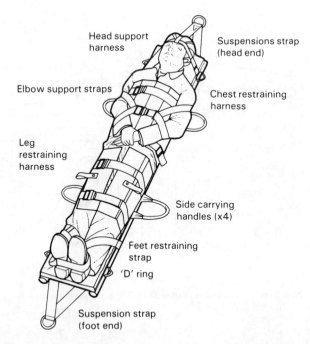

Head support harness

Suspensions strap (head end)

Elbow support straps

Chest restraining harness

Leg restraining harness

Side carrying handles (x4)

Feet restraining strap

'D' ring

Suspension strap (foot end)

Fig. 36.8 The Paraguard® rescue stretcher in use. Courtesy of FW Equipment Co Ltd.

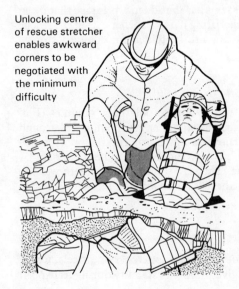

Unlocking centre of rescue stretcher enables awkward corners to be negotiated with the minimum difficulty

Fig. 36.9 The Paraguard® rescue stretcher negotiating a difficult corner. Courtesy of FW Equipment Co Ltd.

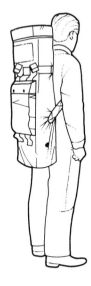

Fig. 36.10 The Paraguard® rescue stretcher folded for carriage. Courtesy of FW Equipment Co Ltd.

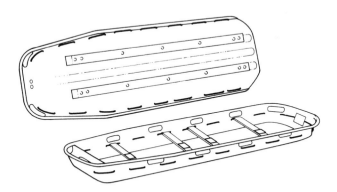

Fig. 36.11 A vacuum stretcher. Courtesy of FW Equipment Co Ltd.

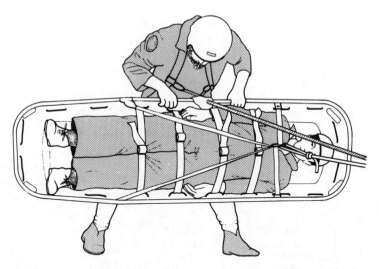

Fig. 36.12 A vacuum stretcher in use. Courtesy of FW Equipment Co Ltd.

As it has wheels, long distances can be covered with minimal effort. The telescopic handles facilitate easy loading into ambulances, where the trolley may be securely locked into position with clamps.

Carrying chairs

These are useful for negotiating steep stairs; as they have fitted wheels, they are able to move easily on the flat (Figs. 36.13 and 36.14).

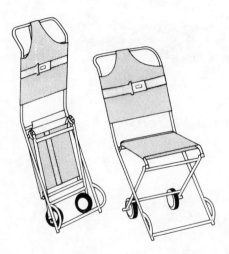

Fig. 36.13 Carrying chairs. Courtesy of FW Equipment Co Ltd.

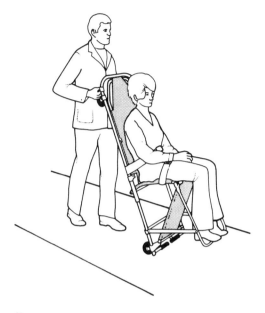

Fig. 36.14 A carrying chair in use. Courtesy of FW Equipment Co Ltd.

Improvised stretchers

It is fairly easy to improvise a stretcher if the general principles of its construction are considered. Doors, boards and window shutters can all be used for this purpose, but more satisfactory methods are as follows:

The coat-and-poles method

Two overcoats with their sleeves turned inside out are spread out with their backs on the ground; they are arranged in line with each other so that their tails slightly overlap. Long poles are then threaded through the sleeves, over which the coats are buttoned to make a suitable bed (Fig. 36.15).

The poles can be kept apart by tying struts of wood across them at each end of the improvised bed.

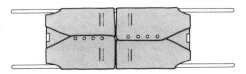

Fig. 36.15 Improvised stretcher.

The blanket method

Blankets or rugs can be used to carry a patient for a short distance, and if available two poles can be rolled up in the sides of a blanket which has been placed under a patient; in this case the bearers must arrange themselves in pairs, facing each other, on opposite sides of the blanket and grasp the poles as recommended for lifting a patient with a fractured spine; this is necessary to prevent the blanket from slipping. The bearers must walk by short side-steps when carrying the patient.

Preparation of the stretcher for use

Ordinary and telescopic stretchers are always carried in the closed position and must be prepared for use when need arises. Preparation is usually undertaken by two bearers and includes three steps: opening, testing and blanketing.

Opening. The straps must be unbuckled and the slings removed and placed on the ground; the poles are separated and the traverses straightened until they lock.

Testing. All stretchers, improvised or otherwise, should be tested before use in case the canvas is faulty; this can be done by placing a knee or foot on the bed and applying pressure, or by asking a bystander to lie on the stretcher and raising it a little from the ground.

Blanketing. For wrapping the patient, two or preferably three blankets are required (Fig. 36.16).

The first is spread out lengthwise across the stretcher with its upper edge covering half the handles at the head end. If the whole of the blanket is placed more to one side than the other, tucking in will be more effective.

The second is folded in three lengthwise and arranged with its upper edge about fifteen inches below that of the first blanket; its folds are then opened out at the lower end for about two feet.

The use of the third blanket will be described later.

Where only one blanket is available, proceed as in Fig. 36.17.

Loading the stretcher

The method by which a patient is placed on a stretcher is called loading, and is usually undertaken by four bearers who work as a team called a stretcher squad.

The bearers are numbered 1, 2, 3 and 4 for the purpose of description, and for distinction when actual work is in progress. No. 1 acts as captain and

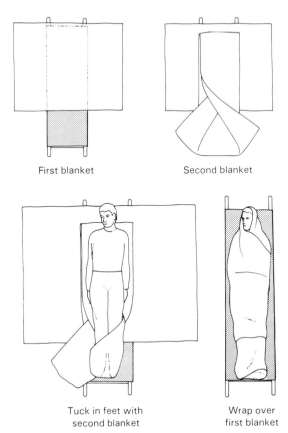

First blanket   Second blanket

Tuck in feet with   Wrap over
second blanket   first blanket   **Fig. 36.16** Blanketing.

gives all the necessary instructions, but each member of the team should be prepared to take his place should need arise.

The men chosen should, whenever possible, be nearly equal in height; if unequal, Nos. 2 and 4 should be the taller and stronger, since it will be their duty to carry the stretcher.

In an emergency, loading can be undertaken by two or three bearers (by alternative methods which will be discussed later).

The best method of loading is to make use of a blanket or rug placed under the patient. First, place the blanket or rug on the ground in line with the patient's body and roll it lengthwise for half its width. Whilst Nos. 2, 3 and 4 turn the patient gently onto his uninjured side, No. 1 will place the rolled portion of the blanket or rug close to the patient's back and then all

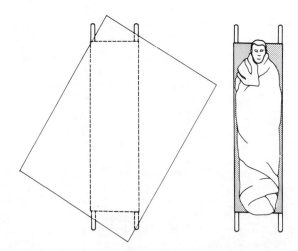

Fig. 36.17 Blanketing a patient when only one blanket is available.

bearers will carefully roll the patient over until he is lying on his opposite side on the blanket or rug. The blanket or rug will then be unrolled and the patient gently turned onto his back so that he is lying in the centre of the open blanket or rug. The edges are then rolled firmly inwards until they are in close contact with the sides of the body. The bearers, two on each side, then grasp the rolls and lift the patient to a sufficient height to enable a fifth bearer to push the stretcher under him. If a blanket, rug or carry sheet is not available, the alternative method which follows should be adopted (Fig. 36.18).

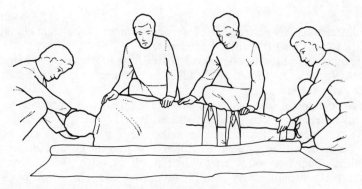

Fig. 36.18 Rolled blanket placed against patient lying on uninjured side.

Alternative method of loading

A patient can be loaded from his left or right side. Throughout this description it will be assumed that loading is taking place from the left; in this case, whenever the bearers have occasion to kneel they will do so on their left knees. If, however, loading is being undertaken from the right side of the patient, the bearers must kneel on their right knees.

Loading involves preparation, lifting, lowering, wrapping, and arrangement of the patient on the stretcher.

Preparation

1. Three bearers arrange themselves on the side of the patient from which he is to be lifted; No. 1 goes to the opposite side (Fig. 36.19).

All bearers kneel beside the patient as follows:

On his left side: No. 2 facing the legs, No. 3 facing the hips and No. 4 facing the shoulders.

On his right side: No. 1 facing No. 3 at the hips.

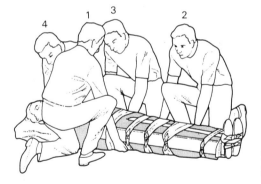

Fig. 36.19 Preparing to lift the patient.

2. In preparation for lifting the patient, the bearers proceed as follows:
   (a) No. 2 places his hands under the patient's legs.
   (b) No. 3 joins hands with No. 1 under the patient's hips, using the hook grip (see Chapter 35).
   (c) No. 4 passes his right arm under the back of the patient, and supports his head, neck and shoulders; and by placing his left arm across the upper part of the patient's chest supports his right shoulder.

Lifting

No. 1 gives the instruction 'Lift', whereupon all bearers gently raise the patient from the ground and place him on the lap formed by the knees of Nos. 2, 3 and 4 (Fig. 36.20). Great care should be taken while lifting the patient to support any part of the body which has been injured.

When the patient has been safely placed on the lap, No. 1 leaves the squad and obtains the stretcher, which he places directly under the patient (Fig. 36.21). He then joins hands again with No. 3 and the patient is now ready to be lowered onto the stretcher.

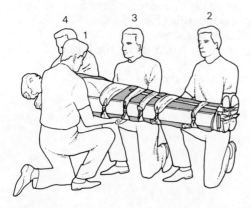

Fig. 36.20 Lifting the patient.

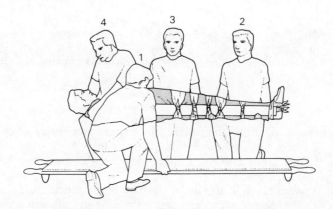

Fig. 36.21 Placing the stretcher under the patient.

Lowering

1. On the word 'Lower', the patient is gently lowered onto the stretcher and the bearers disengage (Fig. 36.22).
2. The injuries from which the patient is suffering are now carefully examined to make certain that dressings, splints, and constrictive bandages have remained in a satisfactory position.

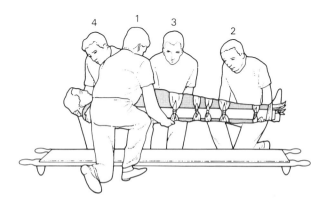

Fig. 36.22 Lowering the patient.

Wrapping

After the patient has been placed on the stretcher, the blankets should be wrapped round him. The third blanket, if available, should be doubled lengthwise and placed over the front of the body before he is tucked in.

The middle fold of the second blanket is now brought up over the feet and tucked between them; the remaining folds are brought over the feet and lower parts of the legs and tucked in.

The upper corners of the first blanket are turned in so as to leave the face of the patient exposed, and the remainder of this blanket is tucked well in round the body.

Arrangement of the patient

The patient is usually put on the stretcher lying on his back, but this position must be altered according to the injuries which have been sustained, as follows:

Head injuries. The patient's head should be raised or lowered according to general principles, e.g. cases of compression require elevation of the head and shoulders.

Care must be taken that the injured part does not come into contact with any part of the stretcher.

Fractured jaw. The patient should be placed face downwards.

Chest injuries. The head and shoulders should be raised and the patient's body slightly inclined towards the injured side. This position should be maintained by placing a rolled-up rug along his back.

Abdominal conditions. Cases of appendicitis, peritonitis, strangulated hernia and abdominal wounds should be arranged on the stretcher in a suitable position.

The head and shoulders should be slightly raised and the knees placed over a pillow, so that they are bent; this position is designed to relax the muscles of the abdominal wall.

Preparation for advancing

Lifting the stretcher

Nos. 2 and 4 now take up positions between the handles of the stretcher at the head and feet respectively; they stoop, grasp the handles and, when ordered by No. 1, gently rise, lifting the patient with them.

Use of slings

These will not be used for ordinary work, e.g. carrying a patient to an ambulance, into hospital, etc.; however, when it is necessary to carry the patient for a long distance, they should be employed as follows:

Application. Nos. 2 and 4 place the slings over their shoulders, allowing the ends, which should be of equal length, to hang down the front of their bodies. Each sling should be arranged at the back of the bearer's shoulders and below the level of his coat collar.

The bearers stoop and slip the loops of the slings over the handles of the stretcher; they then grasp the handles and gently rise to a standing position.

Adjustment. Slings are only intended to ease the burden of the bearers and to reduce jolts and jars to the patient. They must be adjusted by Nos. 1 and 3 so that the stretcher is level.

Advancing

Method. The bearers should walk by short paces not exceeding 20 inches in length. They must keep their knees slightly bent, and should tread with flat feet to avoid spring in the step.

The bearers must walk out of step, i.e. No. 2 stepping off with his left foot and No. 4 with his right (Fig. 36.23).

Nos. 1 and 3 should walk on the right sides of Nos. 2 and 4 respectively and keep in step with No. 2.

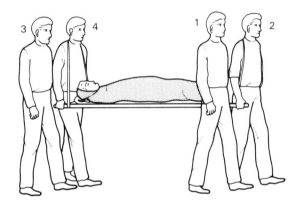

Fig. 36.23 Advancing.

Carriage of stretcher. The patient is usually carried feet first. When going uphill, however, this method may have to be altered according to the injuries which have been sustained, and, as a general rule, the affected part should be carried at a higher level than the remainder of the body. Thus, cases of compression, apoplexy, etc., will be carried head foremost up the hill, but cases of shock and injury to the lower limbs, feet first.

Observation of the patient. The patient should be kept under careful observation during the journey; dressings should be watched, care should be taken that splints do not slip, and the general condition of the patient should be examined at intervals.

Changing bearers. Except for short journeys, the bearers who are actually carrying the stretcher should be relieved at intervals, Nos. 1 and 3 taking the places of Nos. 2 and 4.

Changing bearers involves halting and lowering the stretcher to the ground. A short halt provides an excellent opportunity for checking dressings, etc., and noticing any change in the general condition of the patient.

Shoulder carry. When the stretcher is carried by four bearers on their shoulders, longer journeys can be more easily undertaken.

Lowering the stretcher

At the end of a journey or at a halt the stretcher must be lowered. Nos. 2 and 4 stoop gently and place the stretcher on the ground, keeping it perfectly level throughout the process of lowering.

Each bearer then removes his sling, doubles it upon itself, and places it across the handles in the manner already described under Preparation.

Difficulties during transport

Several difficulties may arise during transport, e.g. it may be necessary to cross a wall or a ditch, or on arrival at a destination the patient may have to be carried upstairs.

Crossing a wall or fence

It is desirable to avoid this procedure whenever possible by finding a gap through which the stretcher can be carried. When there is no alternative, however, the stretcher must be passed over the obstacle.

Method
1. The stretcher should be lowered with its foot near the wall.
2. The bearers arrange themselves in pairs, facing each other, on opposite sides of the stretcher: Nos. 2 and 4 on the left, Nos. 1 and 3 on the right.
3. All bearers stoop and grasp the poles, keeping their palms uppermost; they rise together, lifting the stretcher, and hold it level, keeping the elbows straight and using the full extent of their arms.
4. The stretcher is gradually elevated and moved forwards until the front runners are just over the wall, when the poles should be rested on the obstacle. The front bearers climb over the wall and take charge of the front of the stretcher.
5. The stretcher is now moved forwards again until the rear runners are over the obstacle, when the back of the stretcher can be rested while the rear bearers are climbing over.
6. All bearers now support the stretcher and move it forwards to a suitable position for lowering to the ground.

Crossing a ditch

This is very similar in principle to crossing a wall, and is undertaken by four bearers working together.

1. The stretcher is lowered near the edge of the ditch.
2. Nos. 1 and 2 enter the ditch and support the foot of the stretcher.
3. All four bearers move the stretcher forwards until the head rests on the edge of the ditch.
4. Nos. 3 and 4 now enter the ditch and take charge of the head of the stretcher.
5. The stretcher is carried across the ditch and removed by a similar method.

Stairs

It may be very difficult to carry a stretcher up or down a staircase, especially if it is narrow and there are sharp turns. It is often possible to transfer the patient to a carrying chair or to use a hand seat. Alternative methods should never be employed, however, without the permission of a doctor.

A number of cases have occurred in which bearers have allowed a patient suffering from an appendicitis to walk downstairs or have carried him by a method such as fireman's lift. These methods may be very dangerous on such occasions, and may cause the appendix to burst.

If it is necessary to use a stretcher, a telescopic pattern should be employed whenever possible. This should be carried so that the patient's head is kept raised (i.e. head foremost upstairs, feet foremost downstairs), except in cases of shock or after severe haemorrhage.

The patient should be kept as level as possible during transport; for this purpose, an extra helper at the foot of the stretcher will be found an advantage.

Unloading

This will be undertaken when the patient arrives at his destination, e.g. at a hospital or his own home. The method adopted is similar to that employed for loading, but the patient is lifted while still wrapped in the blankets.

When the patient has been raised onto the knees of Nos. 2, 3 and 4, No. 1 quickly removes the stretcher and then returns to help his colleagues in lowering the patient to the ground.

Alternative methods of loading

When great speed is very essential the following emergency method may be adopted. Nos. 2, 3 and 4 gently turn the patient onto his uninjured side. No. 1 places the unblanketed stretcher with the canvas against the patient's back.

No. 1 then lowers the stretcher whilst Nos. 2, 3 and 4 keep the patient in contact with the canvas of the stretcher, so that stretcher and patient are turned as one. If necessary, the patient can then be positioned in the centre of the stretcher. This is a most simple, efficient and speedy way of loading.

When there are fewer than four bearers, the stretcher must be loaded by alternative methods; it is also necessary to consider the loading of an ambulance.

Three-bearer method

1. The stretcher should be placed in line with the patient's body, with its foot at his head (Fig. 36.24).
2. Nos. 2 and 3 kneel on one knee facing each other on opposite sides of the patient and join hands under his shoulders and hips, using the hook grip.

No. 1 kneels beside No. 2 and places his hands under the patient's legs.

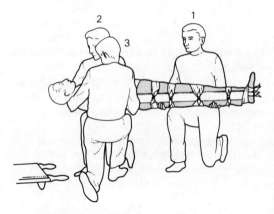

Fig. 36.24 Three-bearer loading: lifting the patient.

3. The bearers rise together, taking special care to support the patient's head and the injured part.
4. They then walk by short side-steps until the patient is over the stretcher, upon which he is lowered (Fig. 36.25).

Note. Unloading is undertaken by a similar method, except that the patient is carried head foremost over the head of the stretcher and then lowered onto the ground.

Two-bearer method

1. The foot of the stretcher should be placed at the patient's head and in line with his body.

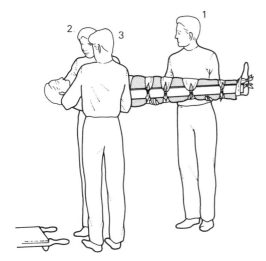

Fig. 36.25 Three-bearer loading: about to march by short side-steps until the patient is over the stretcher.

2. If the patient is unconscious, his arms should be folded across his chest; if conscious, he can aid lifting by placing his arms round the neck of No. 2.

3. Both bearers should stand astride the patient, facing his head, and arrange themselves as follows (Fig. 36.26):

(a) No. 2 places his feet between the arms and body of the patient with his toes as near to the armpits as possible. He stoops and clasps his hands at the back of the body, just below the level of the shoulders.

(b) No. 1 places the toes of his left foot just behind the left heel of No. 2; his right foot, turned a little outwards, is placed below the level of the patient's knees. He places his left hand under the thighs and his right

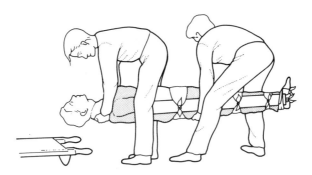

Fig. 36.26 Two-bearer loading: lifting the patient and moving forwards until he is over the stretcher.

hand under the calves. (It will be appreciated that the body of No. 1 is slightly inclined to the right.)

4. The bearers lift the patient gently, but only to a sufficient height to clear the stretcher; they then move forwards as follows:

    (a) No. 2 by short steps.

    (b) No. 1 by bending his body forwards without moving his feet.

When he has moved as far forwards as possible he orders a temporary halt, during which time he readjusts his feet to their former positions; then both bearers advance again.

5. The movements of advancing and halting are repeated until the patient is over the stretcher, upon which he is lowered (Fig. 36.27).

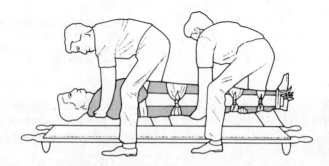

Fig. 36.27 Lowering the patient on to the stretcher.

Note. Unloading is undertaken by a similar method, except that the patient should be carried head foremost over the head of the stretcher.

Loading an ambulance

This is very important duty and must be carefully undertaken. Four bearers should be employed whenever possible, and it is useful to have a fifth helper, e.g. an attendant, who remains in the ambulance as it is being loaded.

The patient is usually placed head first in the ambulance; occasionally, however, he will prefer to travel feet first. This position will be desirable when he is severely shocked and the journey is uphill.

When the ambulance is provided with several berths, the upper ones should be loaded first, beginning with the driver's side.

Method

1. The stretcher should be lowered with its head close to the end of the ambulance.

2. The bearers then arrange themselves in pairs, facing each other on opposite sides of the stretcher.

3. The bearers stoop together and grasp the poles, keeping their palms uppermost and their hands fairly far apart. They rise together and lift the stretcher, using the full extent of their arms.

4. The bearers walk by short side-steps until they reach the ambulance; they then gradually raise the stretcher to the level of the berth.

5. The front bearers, with the assistance of the ambulance attendant, carefully place the runners of the stretcher in the guides of the berth; they then help the rear bearers to slide the stretcher into the ambulance, where it is secured.

Note: when there is no attendant, the near-side bearer should enter the ambulance, after placing the runners in the grooves, and guide the stretcher into position.

Unloading an ambulance

This must be done very carefully, avoiding a sudden drop as the patient is being removed.

Method

1. Two bearers grasp the handles at the foot of the stretcher and gently slide the patient outwards, taking great care to keep him level.

2. The other two bearers take hold of the front handles as they appear, and assist their colleagues to remove the stretcher.

3. The bearers lower the stretcher gently to the full extent of their arms.

4. They then walk by short side-steps until they are clear of the ambulance.

5. The stretcher is lowered to the ground and the bearers take up positions for carrying.

Alternative methods. There are several alternative methods of unloading an ambulance; they are designed to save time by omitting the stage of lowering the stretcher to the ground near the ambulance.

Thus, after unloading by the usual method, the patient is lowered into a suitable position for carrying. The four bearers face away from the ambulance and grasp the handles with their inner hands; they step off with their inner feet first and employ a four-hand carry.

Placing the patient in bed

When a stretcher case arrives at a hospital the bearers will often be asked to lift the patient into bed.

Method

1. When there is plenty of room and the patient is to be placed on a single bed, the stretcher may be lowered with its head at the foot of the bed. The patient is then lifted and carried head foremost over the foot of the bed and lowered onto it.

2. Lowering the stretcher near the bed is usually avoided in hospitals. Nos. 2 and 4 halt alongside the bed and stoop until the levels of the stretcher and the bed correspond. Nos. 1 and 3 now pass to the opposite side and gently slide the patient into bed by pulling on the blankets. Great care must be taken to support the head and injured part during this process; generally there are nurses present to assist.

3. The injured patient, when moved onto a bed or trolley, should always be laid on a carrying sheet placed on top of the bed. Further moves will be easier and more comfortable for the patient.

Index

ABC of resuscitation   16, 21
Abdominal disorders and injuries   118–21
   bandage for   299–300
   stretcher position for   344
Abdominal organs   80–1
Abdominal pain   118
Achilles tendon injuries   190, 207–8
Acromioclavicular joint   206
Adder (viper) snake bites   279–80
Adhesive bandages/dressings/plasters   302–3,
      305–6
Air sacs   37, 38
Aircraft decompression   100
Airway
   causes of obstruction   16
   clearing and maintenance   6, 16, 221, 261
   cross-section through   92
Alcohol
   effect on body heat loss   242
   poisoning by   251
   smell on breath   214, 224, 234, 251
Alimentary canal   78–80
Alveoli   37, 38
Ambulance
   loading of   350–1
   unloading of   351
Ambulance trolleys   333, 336
Amnesia, brain injury   218–19
Amputation   123
Amputation stump
   bandages for   300, 301, 308–9
Anaphylactic shock   280–1
Anatomy   33–82
Angina pectoris   115–16
Animal bites   279
Ankle
   bandages for   297, 306, 307, 311–13
   dislocation of   188–9
   fractures of   158–60
   soft tissue injuries of   205
Antepartum haemorrhage   23
Antidepressants, poisoning by   248, 253
Antiseptics   128
Anxiety states   255
Arm bones: see Upper-limb bones
Arms, slings for   285–9
Arteries   41, 43
Asphyxia
   causes of   91–2
   signs and symptoms of   93
   treatment of   93

Aspirin, poisoning by   248, 253
Asthma   92, 104
Autonomic nervous system   53–4, 55, 77

Babies
   breathing rates of   5, 18
   hypothermia in   87, 243
   newborn   28
   obstruction removal from   94–5, 96
   pulse rates of   5, 41
   resuscitation of   19, 20
   temperature regulation of   87, 243
Back
   bandage for   298–9
   blows to remove obstruction   16, 93–4
   injuries: see Spinal injuries
Balance, sense of   54, 57–8
Bandaging
   patterns of   305, 306–11
   rules of   304
Bandaging techniques   282–316
   triangular bandage   282–8, 290–300
Bee stings   281
Berries, poisoning by   251
Bile duct   80
Biological warfare   269–70
   decontamination in   270
Bites and stings   279–81
Black eye   274
Bladder   82
Blanket lift   338
Blanketing (on stretcher)   338, 339, 340
Blast injuries   91, 103
Bleeding, types of   109
Blister agents   269
Blisters   207
Blood   44–6
   cell types in   45
   clotting of   46
   composition of   44–5
   coughing up of   105
   functions of   46
   platelets in   46
Blood pressure   41, 44
   postural changes, effect on   44
   response to exercise   44
Body splinting   140–1, 161, 163–4
Body temperature
   heat stroke   244
   hypothermia   242
   normal range   86–7, 242

217, 218
7, 214, 221
–51
220–1

8–21
14, 224, 234, 239, 251

est 17–18
n of 38–9
5, 18, 213–14
ion of 18
ssociation for Immediate Care
Schemes (BASICS) 8
hi 36, 37
k airway 16, 17
wn fat 87
ruises 123
Burns 258–63
  classification of 258–9, 260
  dressing of 261–2
  first aid treatment of 260–3
  infection through 132
Bystanders, use of 4

Capeline bandage 309–10
Carbohydrates, metabolism of 83, 84
Carbon dioxide transport 39
Carbon monoxide poisoning 101–2, 249
Cardiopulmonary resuscitation (CPR) 19–21
  burns casualties 263
Carrying chairs 336, 337
Carrying techniques: see Lifting and moving
    of casualties
Cartilage 73–4
Casualty assessment 3–7
Cell structure 33
Central nervous system 48–54
Cerebellum 49, 50
Cerebrum 49, 50
Cervical splint 193, 199, 200
Cheek bone 61, 226
  fracture of 227
Chemical agents 268–9
Chemicals
  eye injuries caused by 274
  poisoning and burns caused by 250, 263,
    269
Chest injuries 6, 95–7, 103
  bandages for 297–8, 299–300
  signs and symptoms 6, 97
  stretcher position for 344
  treatment 97, 98
Cheyne–Stokes respiration (of unconscious
    person) 220
Childbirth 25–30
  breech delivery 29–30

contractions 25
cutting of cord 29
delivery of baby 27–8
prolapsed cord 26
Children
  accidental poisoning of 253
  obstruction removal from 94
  resuscitation of 18, 19, 20
Choking 93–5
Choking agents 269
Clavicle (collar bone) 64, 65
  fracture of 142–3
Cleanliness, in treatment of wounds and
    burns 127, 261, 301
Clinical practice 90–352
Closed chest cardiac massage (CCCM) 19–21
Clothes removal 5
Clove hitch 175, 289
Cold, effects of 241–3
Collar-and-cuff slings 289
Colles' fracture 148, 149
Colon 79–80
Coma scale 213, 222
Common cold 106
Condylar fractures 153
Confusional states 255–6
Consciousness, assessment of 7, 213, 222
Contusion 123, 219–20
Coronary arteries 41
Coronary thrombosis 116
Corrosive compounds
  eye injuries caused by 274
  poisoning and burns caused by 250, 263
Cotton wool dressings 301
Cradle carry 318–19
Cramer's wire splinting 161, 168
Cranial nerves 52, 53
Cricket, injuries in 202
Crush injuries, chest 91, 95–7, 98
CS gas 268
Cyanide poisoning 102, 269
Cyanosis 6, 40

Death, signs of 216
Decompression injuries 92, 100
Depressive illness 257
Diabetics 7, 214, 238–9
  breath odour 214, 239
Diaphragmatic injuries 103
Digestive system 78–82
Dislocations 182–9
  classification of 183
  diagnosis of 184
  signs and symptoms of 183
  specific joints listed 184–90
Diving accidents 92, 100, 194
Drag carry method 321
Dressings 128, 300–3
  for burns 261–2
  non-absorbent 302
  triangular bandages to secure 290–300

Drowning 92, 100–1
 dry/wet 101
Drug addicts 7, 132
Duodenum 78

Ear
 bleeding from 275
 disorders of 275–6
 foreign bodies in 276
 ruptured eardrum 275–6
 structure of 57–8
Earache 276
Eclampsia 24
Elastic adhesive bandage (EAB) 303, 311–13
Elastic net bandages 316
Elbow
 bandage for 292–3
 dislocation of 185
 see also Olecranon
Electrocution 91, 97–9
 signs and symptoms of 98
 treatment for 99, 263
Emergency response 3–30
Emergency services 8
 information required 3
Emotional response 14–15
Epidemics 132–3
Epiglottis 36, 92
Epileptic fits 91, 214, 215, 230–3
 aura (warning of attack) 230
 convulsive stage 231, 232
 post-attack complications 233
 rigidity stage 230, 231–2
Epithelium 34
Examination of casualties 5–7
Exhaustion
 heat 244
 symptoms of 14
Expired air respiration (EAR) 18
Eye
 bandage for 291, 310
 injuries of 271–5
 irrigation of 274, 275
 pupil size and reaction 214, 223
 redness of 273
 structure of 56

Facial injuries 227–9
Fainting 44, 114–15, 212, 237–8
 causes 114–15, 237
 signs and symptoms 115, 237
 treatment 115, 237–8
Fats, metabolism of 84, 85
Fear 254–5
Femur 69–70
 fractures of 152–4
 splinting of 172–7
Fever 88
Fibula 70, 71, 178–9
Figure-of-eight bandages 153, 154, 157–8, 159, 306, 307

Fingers
 bandages for 308–9, 314–15
 dislocation of joints 185, 186
Fireman's lift-and-carry 321, 322
Fish hooks, injuries from 125
Flail segment, chest injury 95, 97
Flectalon rescue stretcher blanket 331–2
Foam dressings 302
Food poisoning 250–1
Foodstuffs, metabolism of 83–6
Foot
 bandages for 297, 308–9
 bones of 71, 72
 fractures of 159–60
 splinting of 179
 sports injuries of 207
Football, injuries in 202
Fore-and-aft carrying method 327, 328
Forearm bones 67–8
 fracture of 147–9
 splinting of 170–1
Foreign bodies
 in ear 276
 in eye 271–3
 haemorrhage by 111
 in nose 278
 in rectum 121
 respiratory obstruction by 93
 swallowed 120–1
 in vagina 121
 in wounds 124, 127, 218
Four-hand seat carrying method 326–7
Frac straps 164, 165
Fractures
 causes of 134–5
 definition of 134
 diagnosis of 139–40
 first aid treatment for 140–1
 healing of 142
 of nose 277
 signs and symptoms of 138, 139
 of skull/face 224–9
 treatment by splints 160–79
 types of 135–8
Friction burns 263
Frostbite
 signs and symptoms 241
 treatment 241–2
Fumes, inhalation of 92, 99
Fungi, poisoning by 251
Furley stretcher 329

Gall bladder 80
Gamekeeper's thumb 206, 207
Gamgee tissue dressings 301
Gas exchange processes 39
Gassing 92, 99
Gauze dressings 301
Glasgow Coma Scale 213, 222
Glue sniffing 249–50
Grazes 122

, 109
24

ancy   23–4

–12
3, 126

for   293–4, 306, 308–9, 313–15
. 68
tion of   185, 186, 206, 207
res of   149–50
position in bandaging   315
inting of   171, 172
e traction splint   176–7, 178
ead injuries   217–29
  bandages for   291, 309–10, 316
  examination of casualties with   221–3
  stretcher position for   344
  treatment of   223–4
Hearing, sense of   57–8
Heart
  beat rates   5, 41, 107
  electrical conduction in   41
  functions of   41, 43
  structure of   41, 42
Heart attack   116
Heart–lung resuscitation   19–21
Heat, effects of   243–5
Heat exhaustion   244
Heat loss   87, 88; see also Hypothermia
Heat production   87; see also Hyperthermia
Heat stroke   244–5
  signs and symptoms   244
  treatment   245
Heel, fractures of   159
Heimlich manoeuvre, to remove
  obstruction   16, 94–5
Hepatitis   132
Hernia   118–19
Hiccough   106
Hip
  bandage for   295, 296, 308
  dislocation of   186–7
Holger–Nielsen technique   22
Hook grip (in lifting and carrying)   323
Horseriders, injuries of   194, 203
Human crutch support method   319–20
Human stretcher carrying method   323–4, 325
Humerus   65, 66, 67
  fracture of   145–7
  splinting of   166–9
Hyperglycaemic coma   212, 239
Hyperthermia   88, 244–5

Hypoglycaemic coma   212, 238–9
Hypothermia   88, 101
  body temperature   242
  signs and symptoms   242
  treatment   243
Hysteria   212, 256

Immersion, heat loss during   88
Incident approach   3
Incident assessment   3
Incised wounds   122
Incontinence   215, 234
Industrial poisoning   252–3
  prevention of   252–3
Infantile convulsions   211, 236–7
  causes   236
  symptoms   236
  treatment   236–7
Infants: see Babies
Infection   131
  prevention in burns casualties   261
  response of body to   133
  routes of entry into body   131–3
Inflammation   133
Inflatable splints   158, 159, 162–3
Influenza   106
Information from casualties   7; see also
    Bracelets, Medic-Alert
Insect bites   280–1
Insecticides   22, 250
Internal injuries   111–12, 119–20

Jaw fractures   228–9
  signs and symptoms   228
  stretcher position for   344
  treatment   229
Jogger's nipple   209
Jogging, injuries in   138, 190, 207, 209, 210
Joints   73–5
  injuries to   180–2
  movements of   75
  types of   73
  vulnerable   181
Judo, injuries in   202

Karate, injuries in   202
Keratin, in skin   33
Kidneys   82
Knee, bandage for   295–6
Knee-and-elbow position (in childbirth)   26
Knee cap   154–6, 187, 188
Knee joints   74
  dislocation of   188
  soft tissue injuries of   205

Lacerations   122, 129
Larynx   36
Leg bones: see Lower-limb bones
Lifting and moving of casualties   4, 8, 196–201

Spider bites   280–1
Spinal cord
   injury to   195
   structure of   51–2
Spinal injured casualties, moving of   8–9,
      196–201
Spinal injuries   4, 6, 7, 191–201
   first aid treatment of   196–201
   types of   192–3
Spinal nerves   51, 52
Spine, structure of   62–4, 191–2
Spleen   81
Splinters   124–5
Splints   160–79
   application of   164–5
   improvisation of   166
   principles of   160–1
   types available   161–4, 165
Sports injuries   202–10
   dislocation injuries   185, 187, 205–6
   muscular injuries   190, 206–7, 208
   soft tissue injuries   203–6
   stress fractures   138, 160, 208–9
   tendon injuries   190, 207–8
Sprains   180, 181–2
   diagnosis of   182
   signs and symptoms of   181–2
   treatment of   182
Stab wounds   96, 103, 123
Stings   280–1
Stomach   78
Stress fractures   138, 160, 208–9
Stretch bandages   303
Stretcher canvases   330
Stretchers
   advancing with   345–6
   ditch crossing with   347
   emergency   331–6
   fence/wall crossing with   346
   four-bearer methods   338–48
   improvised   337–8
   loading of   338–44, 347–8
   lowering of   346
   placing casualties in bed on   351–2
   preparation for advancing   344
   preparation for use   338, 339
   slings used with   344
   stairs manoeuvred with   347
   standard   329–30
   telescopic   329–30
   three-bearer method   348
   two-bearer method   348–50
   unloading of   347
Stroke   116–17, 233–5
   causes   233–4
   diagnosis   234–5
   signs and symptoms   234
   treatment   235
Sucking wound, chest injury   6, 96, 103
Suicide attempts   246, 247, 248, 249
Sunburn   263

Supracondylar fracture   147
Surgeon's knot   284
Suture joints   73, 226
Sweating, as heat loss mechanism   87
Symphyses   73
Syncope (fainting)   212, 237–8
Synovial joints   73–5

T-bandage   311
Talus, fractures of   159–60
Tear gas   268
Temperature
   effects of   241–5
   normal body   86–7, 242
   regulation of   86–8
Temporary treatment of wounds   129
Tendon injuries   190, 207–8
Tetanus (lock jaw)   123, 125, 132
Thomas's splint   154, 155, 173–6, 177
Thoracic cage   64, 65
Three-bandage method, for fractured
      clavicle   144
Three-hand seat carrying method   324–6
Thumb
   bandages for   308, 313–14
   soft tissue injuries of   206, 207
Tibia   70, 71
   fracture of   156–8
   splinting of   178–9
Tissues, types of   33–4
Traction
   leg injuries   176, 177
   spinally injured casualties   197
Trachea   36, 37, 92
Transfixion injuries   124
Transparent film dressings   302
Transport methods   317–52
   general principles of   317–18
   manual methods   317, 318–28
   rules for   318
   stretcher methods   329–52
   see also Lifting and moving of casualties
Triage   11
Triage label   12
Triangular bandages   282–8, 290–300
   advantages   282
   securing ends   283–4
   as slings   284–9
   to secure dressings   290–300
   uses listed   282
Triangular slings   287–9
Trochanteric fractures   152, 153
Tubular gauze bandaging   303, 311, 312
Tulle gras dressings   302
Two-hand seat carrying method   322–3, 324

Ulna   67
   fracture of   147, 148
Unconscious casualties, treatment of   4,
      215–16

ex 359

—40
212–15

-71
–40

tion 119, 195
em 81–2

splints 163
n stretcher 333, 335, 336
orae
actures of 193–5
structure of 191–2
ertebral column 62–4
Vertebral fractures
causes of 193–4
diagnosis of 194

signs and symptoms of 194–5
types of 193
Vitamins 84, 85, 86

War wounds 129–30
Wasp stings 281
Water, requirements for 83
Whiplash injury 192, 194
White (blood) cells 45, 81, 133
Winding, solar plexus 106
Wounds 122–30
  burns 258
  cleansing of 127–8
  first aid measures for 123–5
  infections of 131–3
  treatment of 125–30
  types of 122–3
Wrist
  bandages for 294–5, 312
  bones of 68
  fractures of 149–50

Zygoma (cheek bone) 61, 226
  fracture of 227